Previous Praise for Chantal Sicile-Kira's Books

"Few in the community offer the practical advice across the expanse of autism with the same insight and wisdom Chantal does. Each chapter gracefully and smartly answers questions people grapple with endlessly. In her crisp and authentic voice, Chantal provides a work that broadens the understanding and offers many answers to the most perplexing problems. Well done!"

—Edmund C. Arranga
Co-founder and Executive Director, AutismOne

"[Chantal's] work cuts to the heart of the matter. She approaches the subject by acknowledging its immensity and its baffling characteristics. Yet by sticking to a doctrine of clarity and pragmatism, she also enlightens."

—Douglas Kennedy
Author, *Leaving the World* and *The Job*

WHAT IS AUTISM?

WHAT IS AUTISM?

UNDERSTANDING LIFE WITH AUTISM OR ASPERGER'S

CHANTAL SICILE-KIRA

TURNER

Turner Publishing Company

200 4th Avenue North • Suite 950
Nashville, Tennessee 37219

445 Park Avenue • 9th Floor
New York, NY 10022

www.turnerpublishing.com

What Is Autism? Understanding Life with Autism or Asperger's

Cover design by Gina Binkley
Dust jacket design by Mike Penticost
Interior design by Mike Penticost

Library of Congress Cataloging-in-Publication Data

Sicile-Kira, Chantal.
 What is autism? : understanding life with autism or Asperger's / Chan-
tal Sicile-Kira.
    p. cm.
 Includes bibliographical references.
 ISBN 978-1-59652-842-0
1. Autism--Popular works. 2. Autism in children--Popular works. 3.
Autistic children--Family relationships--Popular works. 4. Asperger's
syndrome--Popular works. I. Title.
 RC553.A88S5666 2012
 616.85882--dc23
                        2011037294

Printed in the United States of America
12 13 14 15 16 17 18—0 9 8 7 6 5 4 3 2 1

For all those who have helped Jeremy
become the person he is today:
Know that you have made a difference in someone's life. We are
forever in your gratitude.

For all those whose lives are touched by autism, know that you
are not alone.
We are all in this together.

For Jeremy, Rebecca, and Daniel:
Thank you for being who you are.

"When you've met one person with autism,
you've met one person with autism."

~ Anonymous

"Autism is an important influence in my life.
The hardest part is not being able to talk.
God must have been out of voices
when he made me."

~ Jeremy Sicile-Kira

Contents

Introduction

Autism is a word we are hearing more and more every day in the media, but to those who are neither parents nor educators of children with autism, the condition is still a big mystery. As an autism expert who travels around the country to provide training, I get asked a lot of questions by parents and teachers at the seminars I give.

But many more questions are asked by people I meet in planes, at the grocery store, in the waiting room at the doctor's, and by those who have a neighbor, family member, or friend whose life is touched by autism, and who want to know more. Several common questions they have asked me include:

- "Do vaccines cause autism?"
- "Why does my neighbor's kid always carry a red plastic snake?"
- "Why don't they look me in the eye?"
- "I'm a grandparent; what can I do to help?"

- "I think my child has an autism spectrum disorder. What can I do?"

Many parents of autistic children have told me they wished there was a quick read to give to people they know—the child's grandparents, neighbors, and general education teachers—so that they could have a better understanding of what they and their child are going through. I wrote this book for them and for others, perhaps those who hear about autism in the media, who want answers just to better understand their fellow community members impacted by autism.

This book was also written for parents who suspect their child has autism. These pages provide a quick overview to allay their fears or point them in the right direction to get a diagnosis, and, if their child is diagnosed with autism, help get them started on the first steps of their journey.

I could have used this book thirty years ago when I took my first job that put me in contact with people who had autism. I knew absolutely nothing, other than a description I had read in my Psychology 101 class at UC Irvine. I worked at Fairview State Hospital in Orange County, helping to prepare young adults for de-institutionalization. I taught them self-help and community-living skills using behavioral methods. Little did I know that years later I would be using these own techniques to try and teach my own son, Jeremy.

To this day I still clearly remember my first contact with a young adult with autism on my first day at work. I was waiting in the recreation therapy office for my boss, and Gregg walked in. "Hi, my name is Gregg Doe. I used to be a sports newscaster. Do you like baseball? Ask me about any World Series and I can tell you who won and what the score was." I was thinking how dedicated this man was to leave a job in TV to work at a state hospital, until I looked at my clipboard and saw his name under my list of people I was supposed to teach. Gregg could tell you all about sports, but he could not tie his own shoelaces.

Obviously, I have learned a lot about autism since then. After my two years at Fairview State Hospital, I briefly worked as case manager for the local regional center, providing information and resources to parents of children, teens, and adults with developmental disabilities. I then worked in TV and film production in Europe, where my two children were born and where Jeremy, now twenty-two, was diagnosed with severe autism. My experience trying to find resources and help for Jeremy in France, England, and then back in California inspired me to write my first book, *Autism Spectrum Disorders* (Penguin), which won the Outstanding Literary Work of the Year Award from the Autism Society of America in 2005.

Despite my personal and professional experience, and what I learned while writing my first book, I continued to have more questions as Jeremy grew older, so I did more research to write my two other books, *Adolescents on the Autism Spectrum* and *Autism Life Skills,* as well as *A Full Life with Autism,* coauthored with Jeremy. I also created AutismCollege.com to share practical advice and information. Over the years, I have gotten to know the real experts: those who have autism and are willing to share what it is like so that we can help those who are unable to communicate. At conferences where I present, I have gotten to meet scientists, medical professionals, educators, parents—all people who alongside those on the spectrum, are working hard to find answers to the questions we can't answer yet.

Clearly, simplifying autism in a short book such as this does not mean that autism is a simple topic, or that we have all the answers. On the contrary, autism is very complex because it is a spectrum, and because there is a lot we don't know about autism. This book is intended to inform, not to prescribe a particular treatment or course of action. Please be advised that this book is not intended as medical advice or advice for treating someone with an autism spectrum disorder. Any decisions in regards to caring for your child or someone else with autism should be discussed with a medical professional you trust.

In the autism community, I am known for the positive and practical information I provide to parents and educators. Here in this book are forty-one little nuggets of knowledge I hope will provide you with a greater understanding of your neighbor, your newly diagnosed child, your relative, your friend, or just the person you pass on the street every day.

What is autism, and why is it called a spectrum disorder?

When parents of children with autism meet for the first time, the inevitable question is "What's your kid like?" because they are all so different. Autism is considered a spectrum disorder because of the variations of autism that exist, from the nonverbal, less functionally-able child with classic autism, to the very verbal, academically-gifted child with Asperger's syndrome. Many parents also describe accompanying medical problems (i.e., gastrointestinal and immune system issues) and sensory processing challenges.

For a child to be diagnosed with autism spectrum disorder (ASD), he must show challenges in three areas: communication, social relationships, and imaginative play. In a teenager or adult, the same challenges are apparent, but the challenge in imaginative play is usually replaced by an intense interest in a particular topic or type of object.

There are differences in ability levels for those with autism; although two people may share a common diagnostic label with those three criteria, they can be as different as night and day.

For example, my son Jeremy, who has classic autism, has difficulty with many self-help skills, has little speech, and does his schoolwork and communicates using a letterboard and assistive technology. On the other hand, my friend's son, Tom, who has Asperger's syndrome, can read and write in four languages, and his favorite pastime is studying world religions. Yet he has difficulty carrying on any conversation unrelated to his area of interest.

In between classic autism and Asperger's are many variations. Thus, a favorite expression in the autism community is, "When you've met one person with autism, you've met one person with autism."

Some children are calm, some are hyper, some are aggressive, and some are "runners," always trying to escape the confines of an enclosed space. Some like to stay in the same spot and twiddle with a toy. Some are very smart, and others are unable to demonstrate how much they understand because of their difficulty in communication. In recent years, more children with autism appear to suffer from gastrointestinal problems.

You may see someone rocking in place while waiting in line at the grocery store or bus stop, or a child throwing what looks like a temper tantrum in a grocery store. You may know a quiet teenager considered nerdy, or have a neighbor who sometimes flicks his fingers in front of his face while walking. All of these could be different manifestations of an autism spectrum disorder.

Autism is a spectrum, which means that there are many
differences in how people with autism behave and communicate.

Is there really more autism now?

A decade ago, it was relatively rare to run into anyone who knew a child or teen with autism. Now, it seems like everyone has a friend or relative whose life is impacted by autism in one way or another. So are there really more children and teens with autism, or are we just becoming more aware of them? This is one of the questions often debated among autism experts.

For many years autism was considered rare, estimated to be present in 5 out of 10,000 children. However, since the early 1990s, the rate of autism has increased dramatically. In 2007, the Centers for Disease Control (CDC) reported that 1 in 150 children were diagnosed with autism. In October 2009, a report from the U.S. Department of Health and Human Services placed the diagnosis rate at 1 out of every 91 children—one percent of American children.

When the rate of autism began to rise dramatically in the 1990s, some experts believed that the increase was due to better diagnosing by doctors and expanding the diagnosis to include Asperger's syndrome in the mid-90s. Many of these figures on autism are quoted from the California Department of Developmental Services (DDS) because of the strict record-keeping required by state law, allowing local regional centers to receive necessary funds for providing services to developmentally disabled individuals.

In March 1999, the California legislature, surprised and concerned about a 210 percent increase in persons with an autism spectrum disorder between 1987 and 1998, commissioned the University of California's M.I.N.D. Institute (Medical Investigation of Neurodevelopmental Disorders) to investigate these findings. Dr. Robert S. Byrd and his colleagues conducted a study and reported back with startling results: the huge increase could not be explained by changes in the criteria used to diagnose autism, by an increase of the number of children with autism moving into the state, or by statistical anomalies. Dr. Byrd's study clearly showed that there was a huge increase in autism in California for some unknown reason. He also noted that parents of the younger group of children in the study reported that their child had gastrointestinal symptoms in their first fifteen months.

The figure of 1 out of every 91 children reported in October 2009 by the U.S. Department of Health and Human Services is a fifty percent increase from the figures released two years earlier. However, Dr. Thomas Insel, Director of the National Institute of Mental Health, said that it was unclear from the new findings whether more children were affected, or if there had been changes in the ability to detect autism. Nonetheless, all sides seem to agree that autism is an important issue that requires immediate attention.

There has been another interesting change in autism diagnosis. According to the Autism Research Institute, regressive autism cases, in which a baby develops normally and then loses acquired skills during its second year, have recently outnumbered early-onset cases by about 5 to 1, which contrasts with the 1950s, 60s, and 70s, when regressive autism cases were almost unheard of.

Lately there has been more discussion about gender differences in autism. Past diagnosis rates showed that boys with autism outnumbered girls by about four to one. However, currently, some experts believe that some girls with autism are misdiagnosed, perhaps with bipolar disorder or with a learning disability. They believe that the actual rate of autism in females is higher than previously accounted for.

Another troubling statistic relates to the age of those diagnosed with autism. In October 2009 in California, about eighty percent of the people identified as having an autism spectrum disorder were eighteen years old or under. Thus, there is uncertainty about how these children and teens will live as adults and concern that we are not preparing them adequately for adulthood; and that we do not have nearly enough structures in place to provide for those who need support. This is a concern shared around the nation, and many federal, state, and nonprofit autism organizations are working together on how best to help prepare for the needs of autistic youth who will soon be adults.

Even if you've never met a child, teen, or adult on the autism spectrum, you've got plenty of reason to care about autism—if not just out of compassion for them and their families, then certainly for concern over the cost to all of us, the taxpayers.

Both autism and awareness about ASDs are more prevalent than ever before, and the federal government has declared autism an urgent public health priority.

Do vaccines cause autism? If not, what does?

The questions in regard to a possible connection between vaccines and autism is one of the most hotly debated questions in the autism community, in the medical profession, and in the media. Occasionally, there are new and conflicting results from research studies reported in the media. One day you may read about a study that positively proves there is no connection between autism and vaccines; two weeks later, another research study positively proves there is. For a complete understanding of this question, it is necessary to read all the original studies from start to finish. Often, only part of the findings is reported in the press, thus distorting what the results actually mean.

On one side are pharmaceutical companies and the government stating that their vaccines are safe, and on the other are parents who can describe to you and show you before-and-after photos and videos that show the changes in their child after being vaccinated.

The hard and fast answer to the vaccine question is this: Vaccines in and of themselves do not cause autism, or all vaccinated children would be autistic. However, the number of vaccines now recommended or required has risen dramatically since the early nineties, as has the number of vaccines given in one shot (sometimes as many as five). Many in the autism community believe this increase in vaccinations given to babies and toddlers is linked to the increase in regressive type autism over the last two decades. For babies who have a compromised or weakened immune system, this increase in vaccinations could be a problem.

Over the years, many studies have been published on the causes of autism. Many autism experts believe that the disorder is caused by a genetic predisposition with an environmental factor that comes into play. The environmental factor could be vaccines, mercury, fire retardant, diet (such as an allergy to gluten, found in wheat, or to casein, found in milk), environmental pollutants, something the mother was exposed to while pregnant, lack of oxygen at birth, and so on.

Other experts believe that the brain is wired differently for people with Asperger's syndrome than those without it. There are a number of findings regarding these differences in brain activity, but not all are in agreement with each other.

Many experts believe that autism is not one disorder, but that there are different "autisms." Autism is diagnosed by observing behavioral symptoms, such as challenges in social behavior, communication, and obsessive behaviors or interests, so perhaps these symptoms are manifestations of different disorders.

Not all children with autism develop in the same way. For example, my son never reached his developmental milestones as a child and had to have physical therapy to learn how to sit up on his own, crawl, and walk. By age two, he only spoke two words. He would spin the same toy over and over if left to his own devices. He never reached out towards other children when in group situations. Jeremy still looks very much like he has a movement disorder: he has difficulty initiating and stopping movements, and all physical activities are challenging for him. Over time, he has learned how to point to letters on a letterboard or type on a keyboard to express himself and to do his schoolwork.

Another child I know who also has the label of autism hit all his developmental milestones as a baby, but never slept through the night and had chronic diarrhea. Around eighteen months, he began to stop speaking, started lining up toys over and over, and stopped initiating social interaction with his parents or siblings. As a toddler, he was very active and had a hard time staying still for any amount of time. Turns out, this child was highly allergic to gluten and casein, among other things, which is why he displayed autistic behaviors. With a strict diet, the addition of dietary supplements, and other interventions, his behavior has changed dramatically, and most of his symptoms are greatly reduced.

My son and the other child may share the same label of autism, but the onset and observable symptoms are different, although the challenges are in the same areas of communication, social relationships, and imaginative play.

The only thing known for sure as to the causes of autism is that it is not caught by osmosis, and it is not caused by bad parenting. For those parents or parents-to-be who are concerned about the possible connection between vaccines and autism and would like some guidelines in regards to reducing any possible risk, visit http://www.tacanow.org/family-resources/dan-vaccination-protocols. Also, when looking for a pediatrician or doctor for your baby, it is important to find one who understands your misgivings.

For a more complete look at the history and causes of autism, read *Autism Spectrum Disorders* (Penguin). More information on this book can be found at http://www.chantalsicile-kira.com/books/autism-spectrum-disorders.

There appears to be different causes for autism. Vaccines could be one of the environmental factors that triggers an existing genetic predisposition to autism.

What are the diagnostic criteria for autism spectrum disorders?

Autism is a diagnosis shared by babies, children, and adults who may all act and look differently but who have challenges in the same three areas: communication, social interactions, and imaginative play or thought. A diagnosis is made by observing those behavioral characteristics, but autism is not always easy to identify because there are no unusual physical characteristics shared by those in the spectrum, and there is a wide range of abilities and disabilities.

Often, autism is described as an "invisible disability" because it can't be seen it on someone's face, and there are no shared physical characteristics as there are in, for example, Down syndrome.

A diagnosis of an autism spectrum disorder is based on criteria set forth in the *Diagnostic and Statistical Manual of Mental Disorders* (DSM) published by the American Psychiatric Association. The DSM is used in the United States by clinicians, researchers, psychiatric drug regulation agencies, health insurance companies, pharmaceutical companies, and policymakers. In 2013, the fifth edition, or DSM V, will be published, and may include changes to the diagnostic criteria.

Right now, there is no medical test that can be given to see if someone has autism. However, for babies or toddlers, the mom often senses or notices that something is wrong. Perhaps the baby cries nonstop or becomes stiff when mom tries to pick her up. Perhaps the baby never coos or stretches out her arms for mom or dad to pick her up. Maybe mom notices that the little guy is not reaching his developmental milestones—in my case, my son rolled over once at nine months and never did it again, and he could not sit up with his back straight at twelve months.

To understand more about how autism looks in different people, it is important to know about the diagnoses that are used, as that explains why two people considered to have an autism spectrum disorder can appear to have different ability levels.

Autism spectrum disorders are classified as developmental disabilities, because they affect the development of the child. Here are the specific diagnoses in use based on the DMV IV:

- *Autistic disorder or classic autism:* This child exhibits stereotyped behavior, interests, and activities, and shows impairments in social interaction, communication, and imaginative play. The onset of classic autism is typically before age three. Sometimes this is described as Kanner-type autism because it was named after Dr. Leo Kanner, who described children with these symptoms in his publications.
- *Childhood disintegrative disorder:* More commonly described by lay people as regressive autism, this disorder is characterized by the child hitting all the developmental milestones, such as age-appropriate verbal and nonverbal communication skills, play skills, and adaptive behaviors for the first two years, then he or she shows a significant loss of previously acquired skills.
- *Rett's disorder:* This is a progressive disorder seen only in girls. There is a period of normal development through the first five months and then a loss of previously acquired skills. There is a loss of purposeful use of hands that is re-

placed by handwringing; a severe psychomotor delay; and a poorly coordinated gait. It is now possible to test for this genetic disorder using a genetic blood test.

- *Asperger's syndrome:* A person with Asperger's tests in the range of average to above average intelligence and has no general delay in language. However, this child, teen, or adult will show difficulties in social interactions, difficulty in using social cues such as body language, and often has a special interest that he is passionate about. It is possible for a person to be diagnosed later in life as a teenager or adult although the difficulties had been apparent earlier. It is only since the mid-1990s that Asperger's has become more recognized by the medical profession. Asperger's syndrome is named after Dr. Hans Asperger, who described these types of children in his doctoral thesis.
- *Pervasive developmental disorder not otherwise specified (atypical autism):* PDD-NOS is often called the "alphabet soup" diagnosis by medical professionals who treat children with autism because of all the letters in the acronym and because this is the diagnosis given to children when they do not meet the criteria to fit into any diagnosis above. Those with PDD-NOS have a severe and pervasive impairment in specified behaviors.

The diagnostic criteria is set by the DSM, and a diagnosis is made by observing behavioral characteristics in three areas: communication, social interactions, and imaginative play or thought.

What is sensory processing disorder, and how is it related to autism?

Although a sensory processing disorder is not considered a qualifying characteristic for a diagnosis of autism, I have yet to meet a person on the autism spectrum who does not have a challenge in this area. When I interviewed adults and teenagers of different ability levels for my book *Autism Life Skills,* most of them stated sensory processing challenges as their number-one difficulty, regardless of where they were on the spectrum. They conveyed that sensory processing was the most frustrating area they struggled in as children, and this impacted every aspect of their lives, including relationships, communication, self-awareness, and safety.

Sensory processing disorder (SPD) is a neurological disorder that causes difficulties with processing information from the five senses—vision, auditory, touch, olfaction, and taste—as well as from the sense of movement (vestibular system) and the positional sense (proprioception). Unlike those who suffer from blindness or deafness, those with SPD receive sensory information; however, that information is processed abnormally by the brain in way that causes distress, discomfort, and confusion.

Babies and toddlers learn about the new world around them by using their senses, then they start putting meaning to what they are hearing, seeing, tasting, smelling, and touching. It is also necessary for them to have the lesser-known senses related to balance and body position: vestibular, where heads and bodies are in relation to the earth's surface, and proprioceptive, where a certain body part is and how it is moving. If these are not working properly and are not in sync, children acquire a distorted view of the world around them and also of themselves.

Most parents and educators are familiar with how auditory and visual processing challenges can affect learning in the classroom. Yet, for many, sensory-processing difficulties are a lot more complicated and far-reaching than that. For example, Brian King, Ph.D., a licensed clinical social worker who has Asperger's, explained that body and spatial awareness are difficult for him because the part of his brain that determines where his body is in space (proprioception) does not communicate with his vision. This means that when he walks, he has to look at the ground because otherwise he would lose his sense of balance.

Temple Grandin, Ph.D. (*Thinking in Pictures, Animals in Translation*), is an animal scientist and successful livestock handling equipment designer. Temple designed and built a deep-touch pressure device, a "squeeze machine," when she was a teenager because she needed the deep pressure to overcome problems of oversensitivity to touch, and it helped her cope with feelings of nervousness.

Donna Williams, Ph.D., best-selling author, artist, and musician, had extreme sensory processing challenges as a child that still exist to a lesser degree. Donna talks about a sensation in her stomach area, but not knowing whether she is hungry or her bladder is full. Other adults mentioned that they share the same challenge, especially when experiencing sensory overload in crowded areas. They shared that they set their cell phones to ring every two hours to prompt them to use the restroom in order to avoid a potentially embarrassing situation.

Many adults on the spectrum find it difficult to tolerate social situations. Meeting a new person can be overwhelming—a different voice, a different smell, and a different visual stimulus—meaning that difficulties with social relationships are not due just to communication but are about the total sensory processing experience. This could explain why a student can learn effectively or communicate with a familiar teacher or paraprofessional, but not a new one.

Difficulties shared to varying degrees include:

- Being mono-channel, or processing only one sense at a time. This means, for example, that if someone is listening and processing the incoming information through their auditory sense, they cannot simultaneously "see," or process whatever they are looking at.
- Being overly sensitive to noise. A baby or toddler may not respond to voices and other sounds or cover his ears every time there is a sound. Parents or the doctor may think the child is deaf and request hearing assessment. Other challenges include the inability to filter what is being heard so that if a person is being spoken to, she is unable to focus just on the voice because she hears all the background noise (i.e., the hum of the refrigerator) at the same level.
- Lights (especially fluorescents) being so bright they may become painful. This affects the visual processing of what someone is looking at in that she may not see the whole picture, but pieces—similar to a Picasso portrait. A child may look intently at a book cover but see only a tiny flower in the grass and not the whole farmhouse setting.
- The feel of anything on the skin being irritating to the point that it can feel like sandpaper. Clothing, tags, socks, and shoes can be unbearable; others may be able to tolerate only loose clothing made of really soft cotton. Brushing up

against another person in the street or school hallways can be excruciating.

- A heightened sense of smell. Smelling something unpleasant and strong with no knowledge of what it is or where it is coming from can be very scary.
- Overactive taste buds or underactive taste buds, which can create challenges in getting a child to eat. Add to that the inability to tolerate certain foods because of sensitivity to texture in their mouths, and you can imagine why many start out as picky eaters.
- Having challenges in coordination and motor-planning tasks in one area, such as tying shoes or playing sports. This is common in children.
- Experiencing sensory overload when there are too many sensory challenges at once. This can result in a behavioral meltdown, perhaps running away to escape, throwing a tantrum, or extreme rocking and self-stimulatory behavior.
- Seeing detail but having difficulty seeing the whole. First example, someone may see the eyes, nose, and mouth but not the whole face.
- Craving spinning or rocking; balance has to do with the vestibular system.
- Not having awareness of where they are spatially and needing to look constantly at the ground to maintain balance, even when walking. This is common in adults.
- Problems in areas such as social relationships, in large part due to poor sensory processing.

Sensory processing challenges affect everyone on the autism spectrum to varying degrees, and affect their everyday lives.

I think my child has an autism spectrum disorder. What can I do?

Getting the right diagnosis is important in order to find the right resources and have access to services. Early intervention is the best intervention, so being diagnosed as early as possible is essential.

Although diagnosis rates of autism have increased, not all medical professionals are aware of the signs of autism at different ends of the spectrum. The difficulty is that there is no medical test that can be given to determine whether a person has autism.

Often a mother is the one who discovers something is wrong because she notices her baby is not going through developmental milestones at the usual pace. A pediatrician who is not very knowledgeable about autism may tell her to wait a few months and come back, saying that boys don't always develop as quickly as girls. However, what ASDs look like at different ages and different places on the spectrum is variable. Thus, choosing the right professional is important.

In the past, many children, teens, and adults with Asperger's syndrome (AS) were misdiagnosed as having mental illnesses or learning disabilities, thus impeding their access to information and strategies that would be most helpful to them.

It is important when getting assessments for a child or teen for possible diagnosis of Asperger's that the professional (usually a psychologist) observes the person in different environments as well as assesses the patient in an office. This is because a person with AS may recite the correct answers to questions of what to do in specific situations, but when it comes to real situations, they have not internalized the information to be able to apply it.

My advice: follow your instincts. If you are the parent, you know your baby or child best because you spend the most time with him or her. If you think there is something wrong, there probably is. The important thing is to find the right person who can tell you if your child has an ASD. Remember, in all that you do, you are not alone. There are many people in your situation looking for answers. Take the first step and see a professional who can help.

If you are a parent wondering whether your baby is reaching his developmental milestones, there is a list of them on the First Signs website at www.firstsigns.org/healthydev/milestones.htm. When reviewing this list, keep in mind that some children have regressive type autism—they develop normally then lose skills previously learned. Also remember that this checklist does not include the gastrointestinal challenges many babies with autism suffer from.

To find a professional in your area who is familiar with autism diagnosis, contact other parents in your area who have gone through the diagnostic process. Contacting local autism organizations is also a good place to start.

These organizations have some local chapters that may be able to help you:

- Autism Society of America (ASA): www.autism-society.org
- Talk About Curing Autism Now (TACA): www.tacanow. org

- National Autism Association: www.nationalautismassociation.org
- Autism Speaks: www.autismspeaks.org

If you think your child has an ASD, it is important to seek the advice of a professional who is knowledgeable about the behavioral symptoms as well as the diagnostic criteria—and the sooner, the better.

I think I have Asperger's syndrome. What should I do?

Perhaps you have always felt a bit different than most people. Perhaps you struggle to keep a job, make friends, or stay organized. Perhaps you have difficulty in making and sustaining relationships. You may have Asperger's syndrome.

Asperger's syndrome (AS) is a high functioning form of autism that has only been an official diagnosis since 1994, which is why many professionals are not very familiar with it and why many adults have not been properly diagnosed.

Why does it matter whether you get a diagnosis or not? If you are functioning well, have a job, and are happy with the life you have, then there is no reason to get a diagnosis. On the other hand, if you are struggling in some areas of your life, a diagnosis can provide a framework for understanding and learning about behavioral and emotional challenges that have perhaps seemed unexplainable until now.

The list below contains areas of difficulty where Asperger's syndrome could be a contributing factor.

- Do you have a tough time making or keeping friends and don't understand why? Or perhaps your friends are only interested in you when you're engaged in an activity or interest that you share, but you have not built a personal relationship.
- Are parties not your thing because you feel uncomfortable or overwhelmed? Social events are a great way to meet people and can be essential for business, dating, and even marriage. But if you are uncomfortable because you are unsure of what to wear, don't know how to start conversations, have a hard time reading body language, or can't gage whether you're talking too loudly, then these supposedly fun events can be torturous.
- Have you ever met someone special that you wanted to get to know better, but didn't have a clue as to how to go about asking her out on a date?
- Has someone you are very fond of pointed out certain behaviors of yours that drive them crazy and suggested that you might have Asperger's?
- Do you have a passionate interest in a certain subject or topic? Perhaps you've been called obsessive, but you think you're just very interested in one incredibly fascinating subject. This passionate topic could help you in other areas of your life, if only you knew how to use it.
- If you are a student, do you have trouble keeping up with coursework and finishing a degree? Perhaps you could use some help in getting and staying organized and planning your time.
- Do you have trouble getting and keeping a job that reflects your abilities, even though your credentials look great on paper? It could be that you are very talented but don't have a clue as to how to sell yourself during an interview. Maybe the office politics are something you just don't get, so you are routinely passed up when it comes to promotions.

If many of the questions above pertain to you, then consider getting a diagnosis. If you are diagnosed with AS, you can begin the process of learning to live more adaptively with an Asperger's brain.

There is a whole community of people who know how you think and feel and who can share helpful information. Autism and Asperger's support groups can help you so you don't have to feel isolated and figure everything out for yourself. Through these groups, you may even be eligible for services such as finding a job or a place to live.

How can you find out whether you have Asperger's syndrome? Typically, you need to see a clinical social worker, a licensed professional counselor, a psychologist, a psychiatrist, or neuropsychiatrist. It is important to see a professional who specializes in autism spectrum disorders or Asperger's syndrome and is familiar with this disorder in adults.

The best way to find the right person in your area is to contact GRASP (www.grasp.org) and ASA (www.autism-society.org). These organizations may have chapters in your area. If not, they can perhaps give you names of professionals who would know someone to refer you to. If you know parents of children with autism, start asking about professionals in your area who are familiar with autism. If those professionals cannot help you, they will refer you to someone who can.

If you think you may have Asperger's syndrome, getting diagnosed may help you connect with people and resources helpful to you.

My child has just been diagnosed with autism. How do I cope?

There are moments in time that are forever etched in your memory—for example, what you were doing on September 11, 2001, when you heard that the Twin Towers in New York were hit by planes. The day you receive your child's diagnosis is the same. You will never forget where you were, how you were told, and what feelings overcame you. The difference is that you feel all alone in your pain. Even if you expected the results because you knew something was wrong, nothing prepares you for hearing the official diagnosis, and the slew of emotions that follow.

It is important to remember that you are not alone. There are many parents out there who went through what you did or are going through it now, and connecting to them can be your lifeline. At first you may be reluctant to contact autism organizations or attend support group meetings—it is kind of like joining a club you never wanted to be a member of! However, getting to know other parents who understand what you are going through is very helpful.

Now that you know what is wrong, you can move forward to

find the treatments, therapies, and strategies that will help your child. Below are some helpful tips to remember upon receiving your child's diagnosis.

- First, acknowledge your feelings, and allow yourself to feel the emotions that are there. These emotions may come back, but you will learn to cope.
- The emotions you feel as a parent of a child with autism have been compared to the stages of grief that a dying person goes through. These stages of grief were introduced by psychiatrist Elisabeth Kubler-Ross in her book *On Death and Dying*. The similar stages of grief for a parent of an ASD child have been described as follows: shock and disbelief, denial, anger or rage, confusion and powerlessness, depression, guilt, shame or embarrassment, fear and panic, bargaining, hope, isolation, and acceptance.
- Recognize what you are feeling and try to use that emotion to your benefit. If you are angry, use that energy to find out all you can and advocate for your child (just be careful not to take out your anger on those that are there to help you). If you are feeling isolated, join a support group. If you are feeling powerless, research online to learn about options for your child and which advocacy group exists in your state for the developmentally disabled community.
- Keep in mind you are not mourning the death of your child; you are mourning the loss of your expectations. The child you have may not be the child you were expecting, but he still needs you and loves you.
- Reach out and find an autism support group in your area that can help you feel less isolated and can help provide you with information.
- Find out all you can that can help your child so you can make the right choices. Empower yourself with the knowledge you need to help your child the best way that you can.
- Take care of yourself, just like in an airplane where the flight attendant instructs you in case of an emergency to put the

oxygen mask on yourself before you help your child. If you don't take care of yourself, you won't be able to help your child.

Here are some websites where you can find local chapters with support group meetings, iChat possibilities, and social networks to get support and share information. There are many parents waiting to help you on your journey and share their experience with you.

- Autism Society of America (ASA): www.autism-society. org/site/eServer?pagename=community_chapters
- Talk About Curing Autism Now (TACA): meetup.tacanow. org
- National Autism Association: www.nationalautismassocia- tion.org (click on "local chapters")
- Autism One: www.autismone.org
- GRASP: www.grasp.org
- Indiana Resource Center for Autism: http://www.iidc.indi- ana.edu/?pageId=1807
- Autism College: http://autismcollege.com/
- Author website: http://www.chantalsicile-kira.com/

Here are other websites and online e-newspapers that provide ongoing news and opinions on autism:

- The Autism Research Institute: www.autism.com
- *The Schafer Autism Report:* www.sarnet.org
- *The Age of Autism:* www.ageofautism.com
- *The Autism News:* www.theautismnews.com
- *Autism Speaks:* www.autismspeaks.org

You will experience many emotions on your journey with autism, but by reaching out to various autism organizations and support groups, you will find help.

What do I do after the diagnosis?

One of the hardest parts about your child receiving a diagnosis of autism is that you are not given a road map for how to help your child. When a person receives a diagnosis of any sort, the doctor usually sits the patient down, tells him what kind of disease or condition he has, and describes treatment options. Not so with autism. Because we don't know yet all the causes of autism in children, there is not one prescribed method of treatment. Many treatments that have been found helpful in some children are controversial. Also, what may have worked wonders for one child may be ineffective for another. The only thing agreed upon in the autism community is that early intervention is the best intervention.

So how does a parent know what to do? Frankly, parents of children with autism have to become adept at observing their children, at reading and understanding available material, and filtering through all the stuff that they read on the Internet. Some pieces of advice:

- If there are waiting lists to get early intervention services in your area, get on a list and remind the organization nicely but often that your child is waiting.
- Find out what your insurance will cover. Some states have enacted laws for autism coverage.
- If someone tells you that a particular method works for everyone and will cure your child, run the other way. There are no magic bullets that help everyone, because everyone is so different. To find out about practitioners and therapies, check with the autism organizations listed in this book.
- When you hear from another parent about a method that really helped or did not help their child, take in the information, but also observe the child. Does your child show the same symptoms? Keep track of how often you hear something works for children whose symptoms resemble your child's. But be careful. Just because something worked for your neighbor's child is no guarantee that it will work for yours.
- Look at all the research on a particular treatment. Some treatments have not been researched yet because they are relatively new. Some treatments with no research have a lot of anecdotal information from parents backing them up.
- If you are going to try different treatments, add one new thing at a time so if you see a difference, you will know what to attribute it to. Taking notes every day on your child's therapies, treatments, and effects (positive or negative, if any) is important for understanding what is helping your child.
- When using the services of a practitioner or therapist, it is important to find out if they have experience with children of the same age group as yours, and if they have experience with children similar to yours. For example, an occupational therapist may do wonders with a child who has Asperger's and a bit of clumsiness, but he may have no experience with a hypotonic child with very low muscle tone.

It is important to ask the people you are entrusting your child with what their experience has been.

- If you have a child between the ages of two and five and have no access to services, the worst thing you can do is to do nothing. Get volunteers and enlist family members to help. Have them engage your child by talking and reading to him, and teach him turn-taking games.

The first step after having a child diagnosed is to research possible treatment and therapy options and figure out what makes sense for your child.

Can autism be cured? Does everyone think it should be?

This is another hotly debated and controversial topic in the autism community. On one hand, some parents hope to cure or recover their child from autism, while on the other, some adults with Asperger's say they do not need to be cured.

Again, it goes back to the whole notion of how autism manifests itself in different people, and the different possible causes as well. Some children are very healthy, but others have additional health problems. Others (like my son) appear to have movement disorders in which they have difficulties initiating and stopping movements and difficulties in completing motor tasks.

There has been an increase over the years of children who have regressive or late-onset autism. These children developed normally then lost all their skills around eighteen to twenty-four months. For parents of these children, it is understandable that they want their child back, the child they knew and loved.

Many children diagnosed with autism today actually suffer from gastrointestinal issues or other medical problems. If your child is in pain, of course you want to cure what is ailing them. If you have a nonverbal child who is still not toilet trained at age ten and screams for no apparent reason, and you don't know what he is trying to communicate to you, wouldn't you want to cure him from what is making him unable to communicate and making him depend on others all the time?

There are documented cases of some children diagnosed with an autism spectrum disorder who have since lost their diagnosis. (For more information visit the website of the Autism Research Institute at www.autism.com.)

Then there are adults with autism or parents who feel that autism is all about different wiring in the brain. Some say that it is the autism that gives them their special ability or talent, if they have one. Some speak about neurodiversity and the right to be different, to think and react differently. Others go so far as to speak about people with Asperger's syndrome being further along the evolutionary scale.

My son Jeremy was always very delayed and never passed any developmental milestones when he was supposed to. He can communicate, and so we know what he is thinking and know his personality. Yet he is dependent on others for most of his self-care needs. Do I wish he were a different person and thought differently? No, I don't. Do I wish he were cured of whatever what was causing his sensory processing and motor challenges so he could be less reliant on others? Of course I do! But that does not mean I am trying to get rid of any possible positive aspects of his autism.

Whether you believe in curing, recovering, or evolving autism really depends on your personal experience with autism.

To cure or not to cure—that is the question, and the answer is a controversial and personal one.

What are the treatments and therapies for autism?

Progress is being made all the time in identifying ways to help children, teens, and adults on the spectrum. This chapter provides just a quick overview of some of the better-known treatments and therapies for those living with autism. All the information for available options can be overwhelming, so remember to look at the research as well as anecdotal evidence from parents and the type of symptoms your child shows.

Consistency, repetition, and intensity are important in any autism therapy used to create new neurological pathways. Therapies that are only provided randomly and infrequently do not result in much improvement at all. Good sleep habits, regular exercise, and elimination of any cause of disease are also important to effective therapy. If a child is suffering from gut issues and other medical problems, it will be hard for her to focus and benefit from any educational therapies.

Many parents have had success with a combination of a gluten-free, casein-free (GFCF) diet, dietary supplements, and Applied Behavior Analysis (ABA) or DIR/Floortime, as well as some sensory integration types of therapy. For many, those would be a good place to start.

Here is a condensed overview of treatment options:

- *Biomedical interventions:* There are a myriad of biomedical treatments and therapies, including drugs, diets, and supplements. If your child is showing any kind of gastrointestinal challenges, immune system deficiencies, or other medical concerns, many forms of biomedical intervention could be useful. For more information, go to the Autism Research Institute website at www.autism.com. The site has a list of Defeat Autism Now! (DAN!) clinicians who have been trained in biomedical treatments and autism.

  To connect with other parents who are actively treating their children using biomedical interventions, visit TACA at www.talkaboutcuringautism.org. They have a great mentoring new parents program and information to demystify different options.

- *Educational interventions:* Applied Behavior Analysis (ABA), better known as behavior modification, is the most-used educational intervention because of the long-term research that has been done on this method. It is effective for teaching skills to all types of people, not just children with autism. Teachers, parents, job coaches, and paraprofessionals can be taught the basics of ABA because it can be used in all environments. Specific skills are taught by breaking them into smaller steps then building on the previous ones learned.

  Different ABA methods are used to help the person learn, such as prompting (guiding him through the desired response), shaping, and rewarding (for correct responses). Discrete Trial Training, the Lovaas Method, and Verbal Behavior are ABA-based methods used with children with an ASD. It is important that a board-certified practitioner oversee any of these programs. You can find one in your area under the Consumers section of the Behavior Analyst Certification Board at www.bacb.com.

The DIR/Floortime Model (Developmental, Individual Difference, Relationship-based Model) has a more individualized developmental approach that has been effective for many. The objectives of the DIR/Floortime Model are to build healthy foundations for social, emotional, and intellectual capacities rather than focusing on skills and isolated behaviors. For more information, visit www.icdl.com.

TEACCH is an acronym for Treatment and Education of Autistic and related Communication-handicapped Children. It focuses on teaching functional skills while modifying environments to facilitate the needs of the individual. TEACCH uses many visual supports and strategies and may be more effective for visual learners than auditory learners. For more information, visit www.teacch.com.

Many hours of one-on-one time spent with an effective teacher who has a good connection with the child is crucial to lasting improvements in a child's development.

Treatments and therapies that specifically address communication challenges, social relationships, and difficulties in sensory processing are discussed elsewhere in this book. For an in-depth analysis on treatments, consult *Autism Spectrum Disorders* and keep updated by checking with the websites listed.

There are a variety of effective biomedical and educational treatments and therapies, and parents need to research to find the most helpful ones for their child.

What can be done to help with sensory processing challenges?

Recently I asked a group of adults on the spectrum what we could do to make the sensory aspects of life easier for them. The answers I got included statements such as "Ban leaf blowers," or "Don't rev your Harley near me," and "Add more water fountains to public places." To us, loud noises may be an annoyance, but to many on the autism spectrum, they are very painful and disorienting. The sound of water, however, can be soothing and mask some of the painful sounds of the city.

There are many methods and treatments that can help with sensory processing difficulties, with discoveries being made all the time. Finding an experienced practitioner who knows what could work for your child or family member is key.

Here are some treatments, therapies, and strategies to investigate:

- *Biomedical Interventions:* Some diets and supplements can help in this area. Donna Williams, author of nine books on autism, was severely impacted by sensory processing challenges as a child. She credits diets tailored to her specific allergies, as well as supplements, as having helped her overcome many of these issues.

- *Occupational Therapy:* The aim of OT is to help a person meet goals in areas of everyday life that are important to them. Usually school districts will provide OT to those who need it.
- *Sensory Integration Therapy:* This specialty area of OT is carried out by occupational therapists specifically trained in this method. The term sensory integration refers to the way the brain organizes sensations and input received to enable the person to engage with their environment. Some of the methods, which help with an overly sensitive or under-sensitive sense of touch, include brushing the skin with a soft brush, joint compression, and deep pressure.
- *Sensory diet:* Often an OT will prescribe a sensory diet of activities to be repeated numerous times a day at regular intervals to help the child stay regulated. As a child gets older, he can learn some activities he can do to help himself.
- *Auditory Integration Therapies:* In this method, individuals wear headphones and listen to modulated sounds and music, with certain frequencies filtered out. There are different methods, one developed by Dr. Guy Berard, another by Dr. Alfred Tomatis. Other types of listening programs include The Listening Program and Samonas Auditory Intervention.
- *Vision therapy:* This method attempts to correct or improve presumed ocular, visual-processing, and perceptual disorders. This therapy, which can consist of a combination of exercises and lenses, can be effective to help process incoming information for someone whose vision processing is not working correctly.

These are just a few of some other ways to help people who have sensitivities to light and sound:

- *Desensitization* is a way to get a person desensitized or used to certain environments; for example, by going in an overly lit store a few minutes the first time and then increasing the time spent.
- *Wearing a baseball cap or hat* with a brim and sunglasses can help keep bright lights out of the eyes.
- *Headphones* with music or white noise can cancel out noisy environments.

For a more in-depth discussion of options, refer to *Autism Spectrum Disorders* and Autism College at http://autismcollege. com.

There are different therapies and strategies that can help those with sensory processing challenges. Research the options carefully, and, with the advice of an experienced practitioner, try what makes sense for that individual.

How do I make sure my child gets a good education?

A good education is important to helping a child develop and learn. If your child has difficulties and needs special education, you will need to become familiar with the rights your child has under the Individuals with Disabilities Education Act (IDEA). IDEA is a federal act that requires each state to provide special education rights and prohibits them from taking rights away. It was originally created in 1975 and reauthorized a few times since, most recently in 1997 and 2004. Since 1975, IDEA requires that all individuals have access to a "free and appropriate education" (FAPE).

Every child under age three at risk of developing a substantial disability is eligible for early intervention. The names of the different programs may vary by state, but you can check with your state's department of health, department of developmental disability, or department of education about early intervention. If you need to find help or information for your area, visit the website of the Federal Interagency Coordinating Council (www.acf. hhs.gov/programs/add/state.html).

In the educational system, if a student is eligible, an Individualized Education Program (IEP) is developed that establishes methods, goals, and objectives to help the child in his areas of difficulty. The IEP is developed by a team at IEPs that take place at least annually. An IEP team consists of the parents, the child's teacher, a general education teacher, a special education administrator, and any professionals providing services such as occupational therapy, speech and language therapy, and adapted physical education.

Sometimes, members of the IEP team and the parents may not agree as to how a child's educational needs should be met, and what constitutes a "free and appropriate education" for the child. As a parent, it is important to know how your child learns. Remember that you are the expert on your child.

Also, it is important to keep abreast of educational methods that you can use to help your child. If you are in disagreement with the rest of the IEP team, there are appropriate ways for you to express your disagreement. The first step is to openly communicate with your child's teacher and other professionals involved in helping your child. The second is to make sure you know your child's rights under IDEA. As a parent, you will need to become an advocate for your child.

If your child is entering his teenage years, it is important to understand what his educational needs and rights are in order to prepare for adult life after high school. These needs and rights are explained in *Adolescents on the Autism Spectrum.*

As laws and regulations change, parents and educators can stay informed by checking the U.S. Department of Education (www.ed.gov) and their state department of education.

Most, if not all, states have an agency, usually called a Protection and Advocacy office, that helps people with disabilities and explains their rights in plain language, providing information in different languages if needed. Often these agencies have decoded the complicated IDEA and made it available online in layman's terms so that parents can understand their child's educational rights.

Following are some tips to ensure that your child gets the educational help he or she needs:

- Know what your child's educational needs are (covered in the next chapter).
- Learn about the educational strategies that work best for students who resemble yours on the autism spectrum.
- Learn what you can about your local school district. School districts vary depending upon how they are funded and the administrators in charge. What do parents and professionals in your area have to say about the district you live in?
- In some geographical areas, there are knowledgeable educational consultants who can help. Try to find one experienced with the level of autism your child has by asking local parents who have used one.
- Become familiar with educational options in your area. What do parents and professionals have to say about different classes and school sites?
- Learn about IDEA and "No Child Left Behind" and what the parents' educational duties are, as well as the school's duties.
- Visit different types of classrooms and schools before deciding on your child's educational program.
- Develop and maintain good relationships with school staff, educators, and other professionals there, as well as others in your community.
- Keep good records of any phone calls, meetings, and conversations about your child.
- Keep good records of all assessments and IEPs.
- Do not be afraid to ask questions, and do not feel intimidated by the professionals. Remember, you are the expert on your child.
- Monitor your child's progress and educational program.

- Keep focused on your goal: a free and appropriate education for your child.

Your child has the right to a free and appropriate education under IDEA, and you must learn to advocate for your child.

How do I determine my child's educational needs?

Every child learns differently. In order to know what your young child's educational needs are, you will need to spend some time observing and recording your child's abilities and reactions to her environment. Planning an appropriate program for a child requires documented facts, not just impressions and concerns. You spend the most time with your child, so taking some notes will be invaluable when discussing her educational needs with your school district.

One way of doing this is to step back from your role in the family, and watch your child for five to ten minutes every day for a couple of weeks and record your observations. Look for the following:

- How does your child do without your help? Does she try to figure things out, does she wait for you, or does she throw a tantrum out of frustration?
- How does she respond to the environment? Does she cover

her ears often? Does she look in the direction of someone calling her name? Does she enjoy looking at books? Does she spin toys endlessly? Does she line up objects?

- How does she respond in a social context? Does she share toys with others easily? Does she play with other children or just alongside them? Or does she stay by herself? Does she understand and follow the rules of a game? Can she use a fork?

Once you have written down your observations, see how your child does in different developmental areas by looking at a chart such as "The ABC's of Child Development" on www.pbs.org/wholechild/abc/index.html. Check with your pediatrician if your child is under five years old.

- Look at your child's learning style. Does your child seem to learn better from what she hears or what she sees—i.e., can you tell whether she uses her visual processing or auditory processing more functionally? This is important to know because many teaching methods emphasize visual, but if she is a kinesthetic or auditory learner, that needs to be taken into account for how she is going to be taught.
- Does she learn best in small groups or one-on-one? Does she copy an action she sees other people doing—i.e., does she imitate others? Does she seem to focus better in noisy or quiet environments? Does she do her homework better on her own or in a small group of friends? Can she sit and focus for long periods with short breaks?
- Does she repeat phrases she hears? How does she communicate that she wants something?

Once you have these notes and observations, you will have more factual information as to where your child is on the developmental scale and how she seems to learn best. This information will help you figure out what kind of individualized educational program your child needs, as well as what kinds of goals and objectives need to be included in the program.

By making observations of your child's developmental level and how she learns best, you will have an idea of what kind of educational program she needs.

Why is it hard to know how much they understand? How can we gain a better picture of the child?

Because those with autism have difficulty with motor skills, senses, and communication, it can be hard to know how much they understand. In the past, many psychologists believed that the vast majority of children with autism had below-normal intelligence. Those who were nonverbal were considered mentally retarded, and those who had difficulties in communication were intellectually slow. Now it is more widely recognized that autism has nothing to do with intelligence.

Recent studies show that the IQ scores of children on the autism spectrum may not be accurate reflections of their innate intellectual potential. Often, those who perform at grade level or above in school have IQ scores that show them to have below-average or even mentally deficient intelligence levels. For children to perform to their ability on a standard IQ test (the WISC-IV and the Stanford-Binet), they must be able to quickly respond to verbal questions and have well-developed motor skills. But, as discussed elsewhere in this book, these are difficult areas for those with autism. In effect, these IQ tests do not reflect the true cognitive ability of many children on the autistic spectrum.

Children and teens with autism spectrum disorders are impacted by sensory processing challenges, and these can also affect test results. A student may not be able to respond in a room with bright fluorescent lights or in an environment not conducive to someone with sensory processing issues.

Another reason it is hard to know how much a person on the spectrum understands is that many with Asperger's syndrome may do well in answering test questions, but not necessarily realize how the information relates to them personally. For example, a young man may be able to tell you what he heard in health class but not understand or realize how this information (such as sex education) relates to him as a person. For this reason, it is important that parents and educators observe whether the student really has processed the information at a personal level.

It is important to remember that just because a person cannot talk does not mean he has nothing to say, or that he is not understanding what is going on around him and what he is hearing in class or reading in books. He may have motor planning issues and be unable to respond by pointing or speaking yet can understand all that he hears.

Here are some suggestions from child and family psychiatrist Joshua D. Feder to consider when doing psychological assessments:

- Think of all the sensory processing difficulties a child may be experiencing. For one-on-one testing, make sure that the room is quiet, has few visual distractions, and is not too brightly lit.
- Consider the difficulties of transitions for those with autism. Sometimes, clear explanations of what you will be doing together, what comes next, and what comes after makes a big difference. Frequent breaks may be needed.
- Pay attention to regulation and co-regulation issues. Do

testing with the child, not to the child. Pay attention to joint attention and engagement, and find the balance between having expectations and trying to build rapport.

- Recognize that one-on-one testing may not show a child's difficulties with the same tasks attempted in the classroom. Children with an ASD may have been taught the "right" answers, but their ability to utilize the information may be limited. This is especially true with tests of pragmatic language that ask what to do in social situations. Careful classroom, recess, and lunchtime observations are an essential part of the evaluation.

- For younger or nonverbal children, it is important to observe what they choose to play with, and what they initiate in their actions. This initiation is often the key to finding what motivates them and what can be capitalized upon to help them connect and move forward in social and cognitive growth.

- Projective testing is often not performed for more verbal children; however, the rates of depression and other secondary mental health problems are very high among those with autism, and projectives often provide a way to understand the child's experience of the world.

- There may be a lot of scatter in the subtests, indicating that more refined neuropsychiatric testing may be needed.

It is hard to know how much a person with autism knows because of communication, motor, and sensory difficulties they may have. To better understand an individual, observation of several factors must be considered during psychological assessments.

How can their special interests or obsessions help them to learn?

Many children on the spectrum are passionate about a particular topic or object, and some parents and educators spend inordinate amounts of time fighting these "obsessions." Unless the special interest is dangerous, unethical, or illegal, it is best to take that interest and use it to help the student learn. This can be done in one of two ways: The interest can be used as a motivator to get other work done, or better yet, lesson plans can be based on that topic. For example, if a child enjoys trains, he can be taught a myriad of subjects based on trains, such as colors, math, time, geography (using train schedules), science, and history (using the different models and engines and eras they were developed).

Here are some tips for teachers to keep in mind:

- If it is not apparent, find out about any special interests from the parents. If the child is only somewhat verbal or nonverbal, you can send home an interest survey for the parents to fill out, asking about favorite foods, movies, TV shows, books, games, colors, animals, characters, what she gravitates toward in public settings. What does she like to do when left to her own device? Even taking things apart can show an interest in something, such as seeing how things work.

- Observe the student. During free time, watch what the student chooses to play with. Take a short sample (about five minutes) and write down the items or activities she chooses. Make a list of the top five after several days of observation.
- Once you've identified many of the child's interests, you can include them in lesson plans or build lesson plans around them. One way is to modify worksheets and lessons to include the student's interests.
- Topics of interests can be linked to other topics. If today's lesson is about the California Missions and the student is interested in construction vehicles, the lesson for him can start with what was used to move the materials around to build the mission. If it is astronomy, start with what was known about astronomy at the time the mission you are studying was built, maybe also what the sky would have looked like when the mission was built, and then get to the history of the mission.
- Create extra credit assignments the student can research for and apply what she learns about her special interest.
- If an interest cannot be incorporated into the lesson plans, encourage the student to read about it or participate in it during free time. This can motivate the student to complete schoolwork because she knows that any leftover time can be used to pursue her interest.

Here are tips for parents to keep in mind:

- As much as possible, include or relate their special interest in any homework or special projects. If this is not possible, use the special interest as a motivator, such as allowing her to spend an hour with her interest when she is done with her homework.

- Try to find a trusted mentor who knows about the topic, or a hobby club that has to do with that special interest. Then your child will have an opportunity to discuss it with someone, learn more, and develop social skills based on the topic. Her self-esteem will rise when she can connect to others using her interest.

Special interests can help students learn when the interests are included in the curriculum or when used as motivators to help them complete schoolwork and other tasks.

Why do children, teens, and adults act the way they do?

The sensory challenges described in a previous chapter are the root cause of many nontypical behaviors you may see a child or teen exhibiting. Because there are more people on the spectrum now, you may observe some of these behaviors in your community or neighborhood. Most of them are not dangerous to you, but some of them may be dangerous to the child exhibiting them. Remember that the child is not just misbehaving, and the parents are not bad parents. Autism and sensory challenges can result in behaviors that are not always controllable. Most parents work very hard to help their children self-regulate, but it is a learning process for the child that takes time.

Here are some behaviors you may see and what they could mean:

- Some babies or toddlers scream every time they are picked up because they are super sensitive to touch, which may feel painful to them.
- Some children may refuse to allow their hair to be cut,

brushed, or shampooed because their scalp is too sensitive to touch. The same may apply to gum sensitivity when brushing teeth.

- A child may find it difficult to pay attention to what you are saying. Eye contact is difficult, especially for those who can't process what they are seeing at the same time that they are processing what they are hearing.

- A toddler may throw himself on the supermarket floor and exhibit the signs of a temper tantrum. That is what a sensory meltdown can look like in a young child.

- A child or teen may wet her pants in a store, mall, or other public area. Sensory overload—bright lights and too much noise—can cause a person to be unable to "feel" her body, thus not realizing she needs to urinate until it is too late. (I know some adults with Asperger's who set their cell phones to remind themselves at certain intervals to use the restroom after they leave the house.)

- If you always wondered why that boy with autism next door can't seem to keep his clothes on even when it is chilly outside, know that it is not a result of bad parenting; it is that everything feels like sandpaper on his skin.

- A student may grab his ears in pain and run out of a classroom or school building after fire drill bells have gone off or after the bell rings that announces classes changing. Loud sounds or certain pitches can be excruciating for some students, so they seek to escape.

- A student may be copying down the homework assignment from a blackboard, but cannot "hear" the teacher as she starts her lesson, so then looks lost for the rest of the class due to being mono-channel.

- A person may flap her hands in front of her face, flick a piece of string, rock back and forth, or engage in other self-stimulatory behavior. This is either to help her stay calm or a sign she is getting overloaded.

- An adult at a social event may not appear to be listening or paying attention to you as you try to converse with him. Often he cannot process what you are saying because of the background noise. Many adults have explained that trying to act socially correct in gatherings such as meetings or parties is really difficult because they are overwhelmed with the light, the crowd, and the background noise.

People with autism act the way they do because of their various sensory processing challenges and the difficulties they have in making sense of their environment.

Self-stimulatory behavior: What is it, and what is its purpose?

Do you tap a pencil on the table when sitting in a two-hour work meeting? Do you doodle, tap your feet, chew on your pencil, or arrange paperclips into a pattern? Self-stimulatory behavior refers to repetitive body movements or repetitive movement of objects, and it is something all of us engage in, in one form or another.

Self-stimulatory behavior is common in many individuals with developmental disabilities; however, it appears to be more common in those with autism. In fact, if a person with another type of developmental disability shows a form of self-stimulatory behavior, often that person is also labeled as having autistic characteristics.

Self-stimulatory behavior can involve any one or all of the senses such as:

- Visual: repetitive blinking, staring at lights, flicking hands in front of eyes;
- Auditory: snapping fingers, dropping wooden puzzle pieces;

- Tactile: rubbing the skin, handling a certain texture over and over;
- Taste: licking objects, placing objects in mouth;
- Smell: sniffing at people or objects;
- Vestibular: rocking back and forth or side to side.

There appears to be different purposes to self-stimulatory behavior. At times, it may be that someone is engaging in these behaviors to excite the nervous system because the person is hyposensitive—their body is craving some sort of stimulation. At other times, the person may be hypersensitive, so these behaviors may be used to calm an overexcited nervous system. If the environment is too over-stimulating, a person may engage in self-stimulatory behavior to block out the overstimulation and retreat inward.

It is important to look at the purpose the behavior serves. There are ways to reduce the behavior or replace it with one that is more socially appropriate; however, you will not be able to eliminate it completely. For example, my son likes to twiddle with a piece of ribbon when he is nervous and when he leaves the house. He explains that it helps him to transition to another environment that may be more sensorally overwhelming. However, this is not socially appropriate, especially at his age (twenty-two), so I taught him to carry and look at age-appropriate magazines such as *Rolling Stone* and *Guitar World*. This works effectively—he usually stays calm and looks more appropriate.

Many adults on the more able end of the spectrum described the behaviors as a way of relaxing at the end of the day after having to put up with too much sensory stimulation, or the need to "act normal." Parents report that their more able teens come home from school and shut themselves up in their rooms or have meltdowns. They suggest that if the teen had breaks in the day to have downtime and to engage in some soothing self-stimulatory activity, perhaps they would do better both at school and home.

Some adults have reported these behaviors to be very soothing. On the other hand, some of us parents and professionals recognize the self-stimulatory behavior in the ones we know that signal that they are heading for a sensory or emotional meltdown. By recognizing these signs, and then teaching the person to recognize them, they can avoid sensory overload and thus take a first step towards self-regulation.

Some research has shown that these self-stimulatory behaviors can interfere with attention and learning. However, these behaviors can be used effectively as positive reinforcement (rewards) if a person is allowed to participate in this behavior following completion of a task.

Ways of reducing or replacing some of these behaviors include exercising and providing an individual with a socially appropriate form of stimulation. Sometimes medication can be useful, for example, if a person is engaging in these behaviors because of high anxiety.

Self-stimulatory behaviors can be soothing or excitable and can be decreased or replaced by more socially acceptable ones.

What are the emotional and financial effects of autism on the family?

Stress is constant for a parent with an autistic child, and parents will tell you that most of it comes from dealing with the systems that are supposedly here to help us. As the children get older, the lack of services can create more issues. Studies published in the November 2009 issue of the *Journal of Autism and Developmental Disorders* reported that mothers of teens and adults with autism experience chronic stress comparable to that of combat soldiers, and struggle with frequent fatigue and work interruptions. Researchers also found that a hormone associated with stress was extremely low in families with autism, consistent with people experiencing chronic stress.

It has been estimated that the divorce rate is in the eighty percent range in families with children who have autism. Despite high rates of marital conflict, many couples do not reach out for couples' therapy. Lack of respite is a major reason. For most, finding a babysitter with whom then can safely leave an autistic child who has toileting issues, limited communication skills, aggression, and other inappropriate behaviors on a regular basis is difficult. Another reason is their lack of belief that they will find a therapist understanding of their particular circumstances to offer any true guidance, preferring instead to use the precious time away from the child to confide in a good friend.

Marital stress around the child usually starts when one or both of the parents realize the child is not developing properly. Couples who have a child who does not seek their attention in the usual way (eye contact, reaching out for or giving affection, searching them for comfort when hurt) find it hard to not feel rejected or unimportant to the child. For those whose child develops normally and then regresses around eighteen to twenty-four months, the parents must face the additional stress associated with losing the child they knew before. Consider also that when a couple looks forward to having a child, each person has an idea of what the expected child will be like. When the child does not match the expectation, or regresses, there is loss and anguish felt by the parent not unlike the stages of grief that people who lose a loved one experience.

The stages of added stress are getting a diagnosis (family physicians are reluctant to make a diagnosis on a once-rare condition for which they have no set treatment plan to prescribe); getting services (a constant struggle); dealing with adolescence (sexual development appears, uncontrolled tantrums can be dangerous as the teen gets bigger); and dealing with post–high school (when few adult services are available).

Keeping any marriage healthy takes time, and too often, time gets swallowed up by the autistic child's needs. Many children with an ASD have difficulty sleeping, meaning that at least one of the parents is sleep deprived. Usually, a role division takes place as one parent, usually mom, becomes the autism expert, while dad works harder to earn money, or sometimes opts out. Differences of opinion exasperate an already difficult situation; how much time, energy, and money is to be spent on helping the child is based on personal philosophy, and in this the couple may clash. Over time, dad becomes frustrated at his wife's demands to interact with a child who does not know how to interact, and mom becomes frustrated at the lack of involvement of her partner.

A common pattern among mothers is to wonder what they did wrong—drinking or taking medications during pregnancy, exercising too much, allowing the child to be vaccinated—thus adding feelings of guilt to an already stressful situation. Also, the couple eventually feels isolated because they believe it is hard to take an autistic child to people's homes and are uncomfortable inviting people over.

Sometimes the couple becomes closer than ever, bonded in their shared circumstances. Unfortunately, the stress of dealing with autism and all it entails—the constant and necessary advocacy at school, the fighting for services and supports, the added financial burden, trying to handle behaviors and meltdowns at home—usually becomes a wedge pushing the spouses further and further apart. Overwhelmed, stressed, and exhausted, the couple's communication becomes impaired and even autistic-like, lacking emotion and reciprocity. This can affect other children in the family.

For most families, autism takes a high financial and emotional toll. Depending on where the child is on the spectrum, the needs, and therefore the financial tolls, may be different.

Here are some negative financial and emotional aspects:

- Most children with autism require several expensive therapies. Many are not covered by insurance, or are limited in coverage (although various states insist insurance companies cover autism thanks to the advocacy of the autism community).
- Often one of the parents has to give up his or her job to take care of the child and help with all the therapies, and because of the difficulty of finding qualified help at a rate that still makes it worth going back to work. It can be very hard to find a daycare or nursery that will take a child with autism.

- Many families end up taking out loans or a second mortgage to pay for the therapies. Some borrow from extended family. Unfortunately, there are no guarantees these therapies will work for their child.
- Unless the parents come together and agree on how to approach this challenge they face, it can be extremely taxing on the couple. Besides the money worries, there is the extreme fatigue of caring for and teaching a child who is constantly needing assistance or redirection.
- For a child with gastrointestinal issues, constant care is needed to deal with eating and pooping problems. If she is on a diet, extra costs are required for special food, plus the parents must ensure she has no access to foods she is not supposed to eat.
- A major stress is "negotiating" with the educational system. There may be years things go smoothly at school, and years when it is a constant battle to have your child's educational rights followed through. Despite existing laws, there are budget constraints, as well as people who are not trained in the best practices for teaching students with autism. This varies from state to state and district to district.
- Parents will explain that the stresses of dealing with the agencies supposedly there to help is often more stressful than caring for the child. The phone calls, the having to explain your child's needs, the waiting and then trying to convince someone who knows about autism but who may not know your child (remember—autism is a spectrum) are overwhelming. Sometimes a parent must file appeals to get the help that is needed.
- Parents report that having to explain to extended family, friends, and neighbors why their child acts the way he does is the hardest thing they have to do. There is constant stress of having a child who "misbehaves" according to neurotypical standards, and people are not always understanding that it is not something anyone can control. Because autism

is an invisible disability—i.e., the child looks normal—people expect him to act normal.

- If your child is severely impacted by autism and needs twenty-four-hour support, you will experience exhaustion. It is like having to watch a two-year-old constantly. Respite is costly and not always available. And when someone watches your child, all you want to do is sleep, because you are so exhausted.

- If your child is less impacted or has Asperger's, the parents constantly worry whether something is going to happen that day. Will he be bullied? Will he put himself in an unsafe situation?

- Parents worry what will happen when their child is older and out of school. Currently, the only guarantee parents have for help is at school under IDEA (Individuals with Disabilities Education Act). At age twenty-two in most states, or when a high school diploma has been obtained, the individuals are no longer eligible for services under IDEA. They may be eligible for adult services, but these are not mandated, meaning states are not legally obligated to provide them. So adults are put on waiting lists. There are not enough housing options, and unemployment rates are very high for those on the spectrum, even among those with Asperger's syndrome.

Now the positives:

- You are undoubtedly the most important person in your child's life, and the bond you have is very strong.
- Sometimes having a family member with autism brings the family closer together. Siblings of children with autism are often more mature, compassionate, and understanding of differences in others because of their experience.
- Many on the more able end of the spectrum are academically gifted and talented in an extraordinary way. Others

have a special interest (or "obsession") that, if harnessed and nurtured, can be a lifeline to learning, even earning money for the child or making a great contribution to society.

- If you are active in the autism community, you will connect with wonderful people and create a lifelong bond with a group who understands what you are going through. Together you can find solutions to problems you face.

Raising a child with autism creates a huge financial and emotional toll on families.

What are the effects of autism on the siblings?

The challenges of having a brother or sister on the spectrum can have both positive and negative effects on a sibling. The factors that affect how a sibling adjusts include family size, severity of the brother or sister's impairment, age of the sibling at the time of the diagnosis, gender of the sibling, and place in the birth order. The parents' attitudes and expectations have a strong bearing on how a sibling adjusts.

Many siblings develop a maturity and sense of responsibility greater than that of their peers, take pride in the accomplishments of their brother or sister, and develop a strong sense of loyalty. Siblings of ASD children are usually more tolerant of differences in people and show compassion toward others with special needs.

However, many siblings feel resentment at the extra attention the child with autism receives, and some feel guilt over their good health. Very young children may think they can "catch" autism from their sibling. They may also feel saddled with parental expectations for them to be high achievers. Many feel anxiety about how to interact with their brother or sister, and feel rejected by the lack of reciprocity. Often there is a feeling of resentment at having to take on extra household chores, coupled with restrictions in social activities. When one of the parents has AS, this creates another set of challenges.

Here are some tips for parents of children with autism:

- Make sure that the lines of communication are open between you and the siblings. Knowing they can talk about their feelings and concerns, as well as ask questions, is very important for them. Let them know the feelings they are experiencing are normal.
- Ensure that the sibling has a private place to lock up her things. Many children with autism have no concept of privacy and personal space or ownership, and think anything they can put their hands on is fair game to twiddle or stim (self-stimulate) with. Siblings need to feel they have their own place to keep their things safe.
- Teach the sibling how to communicate and connect with her sibling with autism. It is not easy, and she will not always pick up on this from observing. This does not mean, however, that you make her responsible for her sibling. It is important not to give her too much responsibility or she may resent it as she gets older.
- Make sure you save some quality time every day to spend with the siblings. Even if it is just half an hour at breakfast or twenty minutes at bedtime, they need some of your undivided attention as well.
- Organize an occasional special outing with your child and you, or perhaps a relative—he needs time to feel special as the center of attention.
- Do not blame all the family problems on autism, or he will grow up to resent his sibling.
- Teach the child with autism one or two chores, so that ev-

eryone contributes and that the non-autistic siblings realize that everyone is expected to partake in community living to the best of their ability.

Having a brother or sister on the spectrum can have both positive and negative effects on siblings.

Why are holidays difficult for families with autism?

Often parents in the autism community will joke that we become more religious during the holiday season: we pray our children will behave while we are visiting relatives, we pray they will show interest in their gifts (and not just the ribbon), we pray they will sit at the dinner table, we pray they won't hit the relative who tries to kiss them, and above all, we pray that we will have the strength to politely ignore the judgments passed upon us and our "misbehaving" children.

Here are some areas of difficulty for children on the spectrum and their families during the holiday season:

- The stores are full of noise, lights, lots of people, and winter holiday music that can be extremely overwhelming for those with sensory processing challenges.
- Social requirements, such as visiting relatives wanting a hug or a kiss that can feel painful.
- Holiday dinners where they are expected to try foods or sit

for long periods of time with so many people and so much commotion.

- Many children are mesmerized by the colors and textures of the ribbon and wrapping paper and do not open the present but stim on (become engrossed with) the wrapping.
- The child does not understand personal space or have a notion of safety and so may run around the house or handle something breakable.
- Relatives may think the that the child is misbehaving and may try to discipline the child, not realizing that the child really can't help it, and that discipline is not helpful when it comes to sensory overload and high anxiety.
- Parents have a difficult time because they know there are certain behavioral expectations relatives and friends have that the child cannot fulfill.

So what can you do about the holidays? With some preparation, planning, and information sharing, the holidays can be less stressful and more enjoyable. Here are some tips on how to prepare your friends and relatives you will be visiting:

- Explain the difficulties your child has with a holiday dinner environment, decorations, and noise.
- Let them know he is not just misbehaving, and that he is learning little by little to handle these situations.
- Explain dietary challenges so your hosts don't expect him to eat what everyone else is eating.
- Ask if there is a quiet room (childproof in terms of décor) where your child can retreat for some quiet time to escape the commotion and noise.
- Send them a short but sweet letter or e-mail explaining why your child acts the way he does and the difficulties of the holidays from his point-of-view. They will have a better understanding of why she won't wear a dress or he won't wear a necktie, and why he may try to escape the room as more and more people arrive.

To prepare your child:

- Make a social storybook about what will be happening and the behavioral expectations. If possible, include photos such as who he will be seeing and the house decorated at last year's holiday season. If he is going to church, do the same there.
- Play some of the music he may be hearing this holiday season.
- Practice unwrapping presents by wrapping a lot of boxes with favorite treats inside and have him open them to get to them.
- Practice a handshake if he can tolerate that.
- Write rules together, including how long he thinks he can tolerate sitting at table, and come up with expected behavior.

On the day of the holiday celebration:

- Remind your child of the agreed-upon rules.
- Pack some little toys he can play with in his lap at the dinner table.
- Bring some foods he can eat, especially if he is on a specific diet.
- Arrive early so that the noise level builds up slowly for him.
- Do not let the expectations of others ruin your day. Do what you need to do to make it as comfortable as possible for you and your child.

Holidays can be difficult because of all the expectations as well as the sensory challenges, but with planning and information sharing, the holidays can be more enjoyable for all.

I am the grandparent of a child with autism. What can I do to help?

Grandparents look forward to that day when they will have a grandchild, as the gift of grandchildren is one of life's greatest blessings. When a grandchild is diagnosed with autism, it is traumatic for grandparents; not only do they not have the grandchild they were hoping for, they also see their own adult children suffering.

However, there is much a grandparent can do to help. Unlike parents, who have a full plate living with autism daily, many grandparents are at a stage in life in which they have extra time to help these children. No longer limited by the need to juggle work, home, school, and raising children, they now have more time and energy (if they are still healthy). With their love for their grandchildren, their experiences of life, and the additional free time they have, there is much they can do.

Parents really appreciate the love and support from their parents and in-laws. However, many parents wish that their parents and in-laws understood that they just don't have free time anymore and would love to have some help from them.

Here are some tips for grandparents who want to help:

- Learn as much as possible about autism—reading this book is already a great first step. For more information, read *Autism Spectrum Disorders* and visit the Autism Society of America website at www.autism-society.org. Information geared towards grandparents can be found on the Grandparent Autism Network at www.ganinfo.org/organization. aspx.
- Accept and love your grandchild. He may not be the grandchild you had expected, but he needs you. Accept and love him for who he is, and enjoy being with him no matter what.
- Support your children as they undertake the journey to figure out what they need to do to help their child. Listening in a non-judgmental way and affirming that they are good parents and that they will find a way to cope is important, especially at the beginning. Realize that your children are doing everything they can to help their child.
- Avoid placing judgment or blame about why your grandchild has autism. There are different reasons a child may be autistic, and no parent ever does anything that would leave their child with autism. What is important is moving forward and helping the child's physical, intellectual, and emotional development in any way you can.
- Understanding why your grandchild acts the way he does (his sensitivity to sound and light, not being able to make sense of the world, lack of communication skills) is helpful in realizing it is not just intentional "bad behavior." Your grandchild will get the help he needs to be more in control of himself, but it won't happen overnight.
- It may be hard to see and accept certain behaviors, but remember, it is his way of communicating until he learns a more appropriate way. It is not just about disciplining him, it is about teaching him other behaviors.

- Realize that there is no right or wrong way because each child is different and will take to things differently. Listening to what the parents tell you is best for keeping their child calm.
- If your grandchild is on the more able end of the spectrum, give the child time to answer when you ask a question. Know that while he may not always show it to you, he is likely very brilliant.
- If your grandchild appears normal, don't negate all the work the parents have done to achieve some resemblance of normal by stating it wasn't that bad to begin with. Realize the parents work hard to help him do his best.
- For those on the less able end of the spectrum (even those who are nonverbal), talk to them in an age-appropriate manner. It is not helpful to speak loudly (sensitivity to noise), over-enunciate, or use baby talk. Talk directly and simply to them, not to the parent.
- Offer to spend time with your grandchild so the parent or parents can get a break, or if you have the means, offer them money for a night of respite and then buy them movie tickets or a dinner out. Often parents don't take the time to relax and recharge, which is necessary for their mental health and relationship with their partner.
- Offer to spend time with the sibling who is not on the spectrum so that she has a one-on-one relationship with you. She will enjoy the extra attention from a doting grandparent, which will help balance out some of the intense parental attention her sibling requires.
- Learn to do a specific task, such as teaching your grandchild to catch and return a ball or play a simple game, or teach a simple learning skill that needs much repetition and positive reinforcement. This way, you will understand both the necessary effort and the excitement from teaching your grandchild an interactive skill. It is a great way to establish a bond with your grandchild.

Autism is both expensive and time consuming, so extra money and time are great resources to share with the parents of your grandchild.

If grandparents become involved in a positive way, they will feel empowered knowing they are making a difference in the family's life, and their adult children will feel supported and more relaxed.

A friend or relative I know has a child with autism. What can I do?

Sometimes we feel uncomfortable when someone we know has a child with autism because we're not exactly sure what it is and how it may affect the family. As a relative or family member, things seem to change when a child with autism is part of the picture. It's harder to find time together, and your kids aren't really sure how to play with their relative. If you are a neighbor, you may not be as close as a relative or friend, but because you live next door, you may have seen some strange behavior and heard weird sounds coming from the house.

In any case, it is hard to know what to say, think, or do to be supportive without getting in the way. Here are some tips to help you stay connected:

- If you were good friends with a parent and in contact often before the diagnosis, don't change. Your friend may not have as much time to see you in person, but you can stay connected by phone. Perhaps she will need to see you more and need a shoulder to lean on more often.

- Stay connected by continuing to invite your friends or relatives who have a child with autism. It may not be as easy for them to get out, but invite them to your party or dinner. If they can't make it, they'll let you know. If they can, they'll be there.
- Find out a little bit about autism. Go to a few websites of reputable autism organizations to get some more information.
- Listen more than you advise. It is tempting with all the autism news stories to share everything you hear, but resist the urge. Your friend has probably heard it all. Instead, offer her an ear, as well as some practical help.
- Parents of kids with autism don't need more information, but they often could use a break or some support. Is there some way you can help? Most parents could use respite, some time off. If you can, offer to watch the child with autism for a few hours. If that's not possible, maybe you could look after the siblings. Whatever you offer to do, follow through.
- Every child with autism is different because autism is a spectrum disorder. Ask your friend or relative what her child's challenges are, and what to look out for, avoid, or do to make her visit (and yours) easier.
- Don't ignore the child with autism because you are unsure how to connect with her. Follow her lead and show interest in whatever she is doing, even if it is stimming with a piece of string when you are visiting. Show her something she might like. Also, talk to her (and about her if she is in the area) as if she can understand everything. Even if she can't talk, she could be understanding everything.
- If you or your children are having a hard time figuring out how to interact with the autistic child, ask for specific advice for specific issues (What can I give Charlie to eat?). Explain to your children about your friend's child, but if the

parents have not divulged the diagnosis to their child, then do not mention the autism, just the behavior (Charlie has food allergies so he can't eat the foods we do).

Your friend or relative who has a child with autism needs you now more than ever, and any way you can continue to be there for her is appreciated.

I'm a neighbor or community member. How should I react to or approach someone with autism?

If you are a neighbor but do not have a close relationship with the family, do not be judgmental about any strange behaviors (the child running out of the house with no clothes on) or noises you may hear (someone repeating the same *Sesame Street* dialogue over and over). These behaviors are not a result of bad parenting. Many of these children are impulsive, have sensory processing issues, and do not have self-regulation. The parents are probably doing their best to teach them and keep them under control. Some children are real Houdinis and can escape from anywhere.

- Realize that children and teens with autism do not mean you any harm. Find out from the parent what is the best way to approach the child or teen if he gets in your yard or if you see him in the street, and ask what is the best way to reach the parents.
- If you see a youth or adult who you believe may have autism and is out alone, or appears to need help, use direct,

short phrases in a calm, soothing manner. Simply asking the person if they have autism may result in a confirmation. Do not raise your voice as he may get more anxious, which may result in yelling or self-injury. Avoid making direct eye contact.

- When persons with autism feel what may be an invasion of their personal space, they can quickly go into fight or flight mode. This puts them at risk of hurting themselves, but also hurting others trying to calm them down. So do not get too close. If they are stimming with an object, do not remove it from them because it is probably something that they are attached to, and they need it to calm down.
- If the child appears to be lost and you cannot reach the parents, call the police but explain that the child has autism, and describe him, his clothes, and the location. It could be that the parents are out looking for him.

Approach someone with autism slowly and calmly in a soothing manner because they may feel your approach is an invasion of their privacy. If the child is on his own or appears lost, try to find the parents or call the police.

Do those on the spectrum want friends? If so, why is it so difficult for them to make friends?

From the average person's point-of-view, it appears as if individuals on the autism spectrum are not interested in having friends. Individuals on the spectrum do not show the same type of social cues or social behaviors and body language that indicates to others that they want a relationship. The adults I have interviewed make it clear they enjoy having relationships, including those who are mostly nonverbal, such as Sue Rubin ("Autism is a World") and D. J. Savarese (who wrote the last chapter of *Reasonable People*). However, understanding the concept of different types of relationships and knowing the appropriate behaviors and conversations expected does not come naturally and can be magnified for those who are nonverbal.

These are ways in which it is difficult for them to make friends:

- Many children on the spectrum are good at playing alongside, but not with, peers. They may be fascinated with a toy but not play with it in the way it is meant to be played with, which means that peers may not connect with those children.

- Games are difficult, so children on the spectrum need to learn turn taking and waiting.
- They may be very interested in certain objects or pastimes that are not usual for the developmental level.
- They have a hard time making eye contact (as discussed elsewhere). For many neurotypicals, eye contact is important because if you do not make eye contact, you appear rude or shifty.
- Children and teens may have poor social skills.
- They are not good at picking up on nonverbal communication skills, such as social cues and body language, and this makes it hard for establishing a relationship. Those who are nonverbal may have communication systems that are limited and unfamiliar to neurotypicals.

Many who are verbal are not good at social chitchat and are frankly not interested in it because they don't get the point of it. Often they have difficulties starting and ending conversations, or only want to speak on topics they are passionate about. These tips may help:

- Connect with the child by playing with what he wants to play with in the way he is playing with it.
- Teach him turn-taking skills using the toys or objects he is interested in, and then try some simple games.
- If the lack of eye contact is getting in the way, suggest that the person on the spectrum focus on the ear of the person he is conversing with. To the conversation partner, it will look like he is making eye contact.
- Teach social skills to the highest level possible. Teach about body language and social cues. Think of how foreigners in a strange land don't understand the local customs and have to learn them; it is the same for people with Asperger's, who

need to learn the meaning of neurotypical body language and social cues.

- Teach wherever possible how to begin and end conversations and what kind of topics to bring up. Practicing in a small group with peer tutors or buddies is a great way for him to get used to doing so.

- Find special interest groups where they can discuss the topic they are passionate about at length. For example, if they are into Legos, trains, or *Star Trek,* find a local club that is based on that interest. Then limit the conversation on that topic to specifically scheduled times with the club by reminding them they can talk about it then.

Relationships are important but difficult for many on the spectrum. With help, they can learn some social skills that will allow them to connect with others and form friendships.

What are the safety concerns for someone on the autism spectrum?

As a parent, the safety of our children is always a concern as they do not appear to have a safety antenna built in, and their sensory processing does not effectively work to help in this area. When asked, many adults on the spectrum have strong feelings about safety and what they endured as children and teens.

Many adults remember putting themselves in unsafe situations due to sensory processing challenges. These challenges prevented them from feeling when something was too hot or cold, an object was too sharp, or from "seeing" that it was too far to jump from the top of a jungle gym to the ground below. Even if they learn safety rules such as "Look both ways before crossing the street," or "Do not cross the street without an adult," their sensory processing challenges put them in danger because all they may see is the beautiful yellow line in the middle of the road or a bright neon sign on the other side, and they may run to touch it.

Parents of children on the spectrum agree on what safety issues they were concerned about, including their children running away, getting lost, not knowing who to ask for help if they are lost, and being vulnerable to unscrupulous people because they are very trusting of others and do not differentiate between trusted people and strangers in terms of appropriate behavior. Parents also fear that something will happen to their child, like bullying from classmates, physical and sexual abuse, inappropriate treatment or punishment from teachers, or restraints being used, and that their child will be unable to tell them. Nonverbal children may have no way of communicating, but verbal children may not know the treatment is inappropriate and not know to tell parents what is going on. Another concern as the children grow into teenagers is the that the people in the community will not understand their behaviors and may think they are dangerous, not realizing they have autism.

The parents' fears are well grounded. Nonverbal children and teens are at high risk of physical and sexual abuse because of their perceived inability to communicate. The abuse rate for children with a developmental disability is 3.4 times the rate of children without disabilities (Boys Town, 2001, Patricia Sullivan). Predators recognize the opportunities for abuse: the nonverbal child who needs a one-on-one aide, an adult who requires a twenty-four-hour support staff, children and adults who have limited communication skills and spend their days in self-contained classrooms, special camps, and segregated living and working facilities. Predators know there is very little likelihood of being caught because these victims will either not be able to communicate or will not be believed.

Many autistic adults interviewed described feeling terrified during their student years. Practically all recounted instances of being bullied. Some said they had been sexually or physically abused, though some did not even realize it at the time because they did not recognize the perpetrator's behaviors as abusive.

Some described how their teachers' behaviors contributed directly or indirectly to being bullied. For example, Michael John Carley, Executive Director of GRASP and author of *Asperger's from the Inside Out,* recalls how teachers at his school made jokes directed at him during class, which encouraged peer disrespect and led to verbal bullying outside the classroom. The adults I interviewed shared the fervent hope that with all the resources and knowledge we now have, today's students will not have to suffer as they did while growing up.

People on the more able end of the autism spectrum are at risk because they are not good at reading body language and figuring out a person's intent. Many verbal adults reported in hindsight that they put themselves in situations that made them easier targets to be victimized.

Sometimes the bullying comes from unthinking adults. Nick Dubin, author of *Asperger's Syndrome and Bullying,* remembers how some high school teachers contributed to his low self-esteem and reinforced his own feelings of shame through their comments about his inability to tie his shoes, although he was the best singles tennis player on the varsity tennis team. The teachers thought Nick was not trying hard enough, when, in fact, he was trying very hard but had a very uneven motor skill profile.

Below are some tips to help teach children and teenagers with autism about safety.

- For concerns such as being unable to feel hot and cold, sensory integration therapy can help with some sensory challenges. Techniques such as brushing and joint compression to help organize the sensory system can be helpful. Vision therapy and auditory integration training can help as well with recognizing what is being seen and heard.
- If he can tolerate it, make sure your child has an identifying tag attached to him in a place that he cannot lose it, such as shoelaces, clothes, a belt hook, or a bracelet.
- If your child is a "runner," or escape artist, provide the neighbors with a photo of your child, along with a friendly request that they get in touch immediately if they see this person wandering on his own. You may offer to return the

favor for a neighbor who may want someone to keep an eye out for one of her loved ones (person or pet).

- It is crucial to teach the same safety rules you would to any child, such as, "Don't open the door for anyone when you are home alone." What will differ from child to child is how, and for how long, a lesson such as this needs to be taught. Even if you do not know how much the child understands because he has few communication skills, create social storybooks with pictures covering the rules and situations described in this chapter (such as who is a safe person to approach when lost), and go over it many times in a matter-of-fact way. Social stories that explain why we don't open the door to strangers, and what constitutes a stranger, can be helpful. Practicing skills by having known and unknown people come to the door reinforce the lesson and are essential to learning. The purpose is not to scare the child but to have him become aware of situations and what to do.
- Having even a rudimentary communication system in place that can be used in public is helpful and necessary.
- A school environment that strictly enforces a no-bullying policy is important. Preventing abusive behavior and bullying requires information sharing and awareness training. Peer and teacher training on autism and Asperger's syndrome should be provided.
- Sensitizing the other students as to what autism is, teaching the child on the spectrum what abusive behavior is, and providing the child with a safe place and safe person to go to at school is very important.
- Teach the "hidden curriculum," the unwritten rules of social behavior, to children and teens on the more functionally able end of the spectrum. This enables them to learn what neurotypicals usually pick up by osmosis, gives them a greater understanding of the social world, and makes them less easy prey.
- Junior and high school students with autism, no matter the

ability level, should be provided sex education. Discussions on sex and what constitutes a sexual act, as well as the rights and responsibilities attached, is paramount to their safety from bullying of a sexual nature. One way to begin teaching these important but complicated topics is with a discussion of "private" and "public." Even those more impacted by autism can benefit from adults using icons to teach these concepts early on (this is explained in a separate chapter).

- More police and other first responder training, as well as community awareness about autism in general and behaviors a youth or adult may exhibit, is crucial for the safety and community living of those on the spectrum. First respondents in many areas are receiving training, but it is needed everywhere. Community awareness of what autism looks like at different ages and ability levels is necessary for citizens to recognize that a child is in danger. Often, people see a child with autism and think he is misbehaving, or see a teen or adult acting strangely and think he is under the influence of drugs because the observer does not recognize or understand how a person with Asperger's may react or behave when anxious or overwhelmed.

More information on different aspects of safety, including tracking devices and alert systems, is available on the following web pages:

- www.nationalautismassociation.org/safetytoolkit.php
- http://www.autism-society.org/living-with-autism/how-we-can-help/safe-and-sound
- www.amberalertregistry.com/aar-news/announces-collab-partners.html
- http://www.autismsafety.org

Although we want our children to be safe and feel safe, as parents and teachers, we need to strike a balance between creating a safe environment and letting them experience opportunities that could expand their world and enrich their lives. For this to happen, the community as a whole has to have a certain amount of awareness about autism and its challenges. By providing autism awareness training to peers and school staff, as well as teaching the children on the spectrum communication, basic safety skills, and some social relationship skills in a way they can understand, we can provide a healthier and safer environment in which they can thrive.

There are many safety concerns for those on the spectrum, but these can be diminished by teaching them safety skills and educating the community about safety concerns in regards to children on the spectrum.

What communication difficulties do they have?

Communication is one of the most important and basic skills a person needs to have, but it usually does not come easily for a child on the spectrum. Challenges in communication is one of the defining characteristics of an autism spectrum disorder. All people need a form of communication to express their needs in order to have them met. If a child does not have an appropriate communication system, he will learn to communicate through behavior such as screaming or tantruming, which may be inappropriate to express pain or frustration, but effective.

Sue Rubin, writer and star of the documentary "Autism is a World," is a nonverbal college student and disability advocate. She often discusses the impact of communication on behavior, sharing that as she learned to type, she was able to explain to others what was causing her behaviors and could then get help in those areas. In high school, typing allowed her to write her own social stories and behavior plans. As her communication skills increased, her inappropriate behaviors decreased.

Those with Asperger's and on the more functionally able end

of the spectrum may have more subtle communication challenges, but these are just as important for surviving in a neurotypical world. Some have challenges in starting and ending conversations, or speaking on topics other than their preferred area of interest. Individuals who have ASD do not come equipped with the same ability to understand the "hidden curriculum." These are the unwritten social rules and expectations of behavior that we all seem to know without them being taught. As a result, those with ASDs break a lot of social and behavioral rules without realizing it. This, coupled with their difficulty in generalizing information from one situation to another, leads them to make the same mistakes at a tremendous social cost.

Many tend to have trouble reading body language and understanding implied meanings and metaphors, and this can lead to frustration and misunderstanding. Michael Crouch, college postmaster at The Crown College of the Bible in Tennessee, credits some girls with helping him develop good communication skills. Some of his areas of difficulty were speaking too fast or too low, stuttering, and making poor eye contact. When he was a teenager, five girls at his church encouraged him to join the choir, an experience that helped him overcome some of his difficulties. Having a group of non-autistic peers who shared his interests and provided opportunities for modeling and practicing good communication skills over a few years helped Michael become the accomplished speaker he is today.

Here are some tips and just a few methods for helping your child who has limited or no verbal communication skills:

- If your child is nonverbal or has limited verbal communication skills, try some alternative communication system— and do it earlier rather than later. Research shows that using some form of augmentative communication system (such as PECS, the Picture Exchange Communication System, or signing) does not prevent the child from speaking, but rather helps the child develop useful speech. Having a way to communicate will decrease the child's frustration and will result in less inappropriate behaviors. You may need to advocate for this at school.

- Find a good speech therapist. Speech-language therapy is the treatment for most children with speech or language disorders. A speech disorder refers to a problem with the actual production of sounds, involving the muscles, whereas a language disorder refers to a difficulty understanding or putting words together to communicate ideas. Find a therapist who works with children on the spectrum resembling yours in ability level, and who is knowledgeable about the latest techniques.

- Verbal Behavior has been known to be effective with many children in developing speech and language skills. Applied Verbal Behavior, or VB, is based on the principals of applied behavior analysis and is used to teach and reinforce speech. In his 1957 analysis *Verbal Behavior*, B. F. Skinner described categories of speech, or verbal behavior: mands are requests ("I want a drink"); echoes are verbal imitations; tacts are labels ("toy," "elephant"); and intraverbals are conversational responses ("What do you want?"). More information on these categories can be found at autismweb.com/aba.htm.

- The Picture Exchange Communication System (PECS) was developed in 1985 as an augmentative communication system that teaches children and adults with autism and other communication deficits to initiate communication with others. PECS can be used readily in a variety of settings and has received recognition for focusing on the initiation component of communication. PECS does not require complex or expensive materials, but basically picture or word icons and Velcro, and some training for staff. For more information, visit www.pecs.com.

- Rapid Prompting Method (RPM) was developed by Soma Mukhopadhyay as she tried to find ways to teach her son

Tito, who is severely impacted by autism. RPM uses a "Teach-Ask" paradigm for eliciting responses through intensive verbal, auditory, visual, and tactile prompts. Prompting competes with each student's self-stimulatory behavior, and is designed to help students initiate a response. Student responses evolve from picking up answers, to pointing, to typing and writing, which reveals students' comprehension, academic abilities, and eventually, conversational skills. For more information, visit www.halo-soma.org.

- Supported Typing is a form of augmentative and alternative communication (AAC) that has been an effective means of expression for some with developmental disabilities, including autism. The individual learns to communicate by typing on a keyboard or pointing at letters, images, or other symbols to represent messages. Supported Typing involves a combination of physical and emotional support to an individual who has difficulties with speech and with intentional pointing (i.e., unassisted typing). For more information, visit http://soe.syr.edu/centers_institutes/institute_communication_inclusion/default.aspx.

Here are some tips for those with functional verbal skills:

- Teaching conversation skills may be necessary. To help an individual develop good communication, have him practice starting and ending conversations, making conversation on varied topics, and limiting the time talking about his favorite interest.
- The "hidden curriculum" needs to be taught. They must learn these rules of communication and practice applying them, which is crucial to children and especially teenagers in junior high and high school, when social expectations begin to rise. A good resource is *The Hidden Curriculum: Practical Solutions for Understanding Unstated Rules in*

Social Situations, by Brenda Smith Myles, Melissa L. Trautman, and Ronda L. Schelvan.

- Teaching metaphors can be very helpful. Those with Asperger's often do not pick up on metaphors and can't read between the lines; however, they can become quite adept at it when taught the meanings of certain expressions.
- Teaching social cues and body language is useful. Often those with autism cannot read body language, a real problem in junior high and high school when the social expectations rise. Working on self-awareness, awareness of others, perceived intent, and the rules of personal space—that staying an arm's length away from people is the norm in our American culture—is helpful for social reasons as well as safety.

There are different communication difficulties depending on where the person is on the spectrum, but there are many options for providing a communication system or improving their verbal communication skills.

Why are transitions from one place to another, or one activity to another, problematic?

By all accounts, transitions are difficult for those on the spectrum. If a person is oversensitive to light, sound, smell, and touch, he may be anxious to move to a different activity or environment where the sensory stimuli are unpredictable. When interviewed, adults with autism indicated that surprises were difficult because they could not assimilate the information fast enough. For example, Brian King, LCSW, says that for this reason, surprises, such as his boss asking him to do something right away without advance notice, can make him very anxious.

Many transition strategies can be helpful, whether used together or separately. Some can be faded over time and put back during times of major transitions, such as changing from one school to another, or leaving high school for a job, or moving to another living situation or house. Here are some strategies to help deal with these transitions:

- *Having a schedule:* The most helpful strategy, adults reported when asked, was knowing in advance where they were going, who they were going to see, and what was going to happen, so that they could anticipate and prepare themselves for the sensory aspects of their day. Using a daily and monthly written or picture schedule, and having it available, is probably the most important transition strategy. Using a schedule and reading it to the child with autism (if he does better with auditory processing than visual) will help him know what to anticipate. In order to teach flexibility and how to prepare for the unexpected, include a written reminder on the schedule such as "Sometimes the schedule will change."

- *Priming:* Priming is helpful for difficult transitions, or for preparation for tests. For example, my son had a very hard time with visits to the dentist. At first I put the dentist icon out for days ahead of the appointment and showed him and told him every day for a week what would take place. He needed that time to prepare for the sensory onslaught. If I forgot, I could not get him out of the car when we got to the medical building. After a few years, I could just tell him the morning of. Preparing a student about an upcoming test—what will be covered and how to take it—can be helpful.

- *Cueing individuals before a transition:* It is helpful to remind a person, visually as well as verbally, before a transition will take place ("Time for a bath now, put your math away").

- *Using a visual timer:* Having a visual timer that shows the amount of time remaining in an activity before transitioning to another one is very useful for making an abstract concept concrete. The Time Timer at www.timetimer.com clearly shows in red the amount of time left.

- *Transition cards:* These cards with photos or words representing activities of the day can be given to the person as a useful cue that it is time to transition to another activity, and what that activity is. For kinesthetic learners, an object representing the activity can be used.

- *Transitional objects:* A transitional object a person can hold is extremely helpful. New environments are unpredictable with different people, lights, and noise, so having a familiar object helps a child or teen stay regulated and gives him something to focus on that doesn't require any mental effort.
- *Strategies dealing directly with the sensory:* Other strategies include those dealing with senses, such as changing diets, wearing special lenses, having a sensory diet, undergoing auditory and vision therapy, and practicing desensitization techniques.
- *Therapy for emotional aspects:* For some, seeing a therapist on a regular basis to help with the emotional aspects of changes was a factor in being able to develop coping skills.

Transitions are difficult because if those on the spectrum do not know what is coming next, they cannot anticipate sensory processing challenges they may face. Giving them advance notice of what is going to happen next is the most helpful strategy.

How can we teach the concept of private and public behavior?

Children and teens with autism do not have an innate sense of personal space, making it hard for many to grasp the concept of what is appropriate and inappropriate behavior in public or towards others. It is extremely important that teenagers understand the different behaviors and conversations that are appropriate in public, and the kind that are meant to be private. For example, touching certain parts of your body in public is inappropriate, as is touching other people. Your child or teenager may love touching the brightly colored raised letters on a sweatshirt worn by another person, but he must learn not to or he will continue as a teenager to do so. One day he may be perceived as touching a woman's breast—even if he thinks he is touching the letters on her shirt—and therefore could get in trouble. Having conversations at school that are appropriate at the family breakfast table but are inappropriate in a peer lunchroom setting can get a teen labeled weird at school and prevent friendships from developing.

One way of teaching the concept of private and public that can be used with different ability levels is to show two picture icons, one of a fully clothed figure labeled "public," and one of a figure clothed only in underwear labeled "private." A good time to start teaching this is when your child is getting too old to run around the house with no clothes on.

Show your tween the icons, and explain which behaviors are private and should be done in his room only and which are public and okay everywhere in the house. For those more impacted by autism, putting the private icon inside his or her bedroom door and the public one outside his bedroom door is helpful. Then you can remind your tween when inappropriate private behaviors are occurring outside his room ("That is a private behavior you do in the privacy of your room") and take him to his bedroom and show him the icons. The same applies to appropriate and inappropriate conversations. An adolescent female may need to be reminded that it is okay to discuss her menstrual cycle at the breakfast table at home (private conversation), but not in the school cafeteria at lunchtime (public place).

Teaching the concept of private and public is crucial to helping your child understand appropriate and inappropriate public behavior, a concept that will be invaluable as he or she becomes more independent.

The concept of appropriate and inappropriate behaviors and conversations can be taught by using icons labeled "public" and "private."

How can we teach them to be more independent, but also teach them interdependence?

Independence is a goal we all strive for with our children. It is important for many reasons, and may take longer than expected for those on the more able end of the spectrum. For those on the less able end, we still strive to get them as independent as possible. The sooner we start working on self-help and living skills, the better.

Sometimes too much emphasis is put on teaching independence skills while children are growing up. However, many adults on the spectrum have discussed the importance of teaching children interdependence skills—how to ask for help, how to approach a store clerk, how to network as they get older. For them, interdependence did not come as easily as it does for neurotypicals. Yet asking people you know for assistance is how social and community life functions.

For example, young children on the spectrum do not naturally seek out others when they are hurt on the playground or when their shoe comes untied; that is something that needs to be taught to them. This "asking-for-help" skill when little can then translate into learning how to network as an adult, especially for those with Asperger's who may be living on their own or looking for a job.

Parents of children with autism need to accept that they will be parenting for a lot longer than parents of neurotypical children, according to Zosia Zaks, author of *Life and Love: Positive Strategies for Autistic Adults*. For many autistic people I interviewed, some skill acquisition came later in life, and many are still improving themselves and their essential skills. This is relieving to know because so often as parents and educators we hear about the "windows of opportunity" in terms of age and can become discouraged by our own doubts as well as those of others ("If they haven't learned by now . . .").

Two of the greatest challenges to self-sufficiency are executive functioning (being able to get and stay organized) and sensory processing. These tips address these challenges and help teach independence:

- Establishing routines helps some children learn organizational skills and responsibility, important aspects of self-sufficiency.
- If your child has difficulties with some self-help routines, do a task analysis by looking at what step in the routine is creating a challenge and figuring out why. If there is a sensory problem (perhaps the child cannot tolerate water from the shower hitting his scalp), find a solution (use a big sponge to gently wet and rinse hair). Then teach that step separately, and put it back in the routine.

Make the child responsible for certain chores in the house. This will also give him the notion of contributing to community life.

These are tips for teaching interdependence:

- Teach children early on how to ask for help. Turning to trusted non-autistic "helpers" is a vital skill they need to learn to prepare for different types of social relationships when they are teenagers and then adults.

- During a task or chore, take away some needed material, and teach the child to ask for it from a trusted adult in the room. For nonverbals, this can be done with picture or word icons or other augmentative communication systems.
- In very young children with Asperger's, shopping in stores is a great setting for learning about safety and developing interdependence skills. First, give the child a feeling of security during the first few shopping trips. This can be done by staying at the young child's side and telling her or him, "Never be afraid. I will never leave you. You will not get lost." Then once the child feels secure, he or she can be taught to recognize and approach a store employee to ask for help. This is a useful skill to find things, but more importantly, a vital skill if a child gets separated from his or her parent. For more in-depth information, read *Autism Life Skills*.

Independence can be taught by establishing routines; interdependence can be taught by teaching children how to ask for help.

How can we teach them self-regulation?

Self-regulation is a necessary skill for taking part in community life. To self-regulate means to be able to recognize, communicate, and regulate sensory as well as emotional overload. Self-regulation entails a certain amount of self-awareness. Being self-aware means being able to recognize:

- the different emotions in ourselves as well as in others,
- how our bodies are reacting to sensory stimuli,
- when we are emotionally overloaded, and
- when we are having a sensory overload.

Think about how you feel in different situations. For instance, you are ten minutes late to an important meeting and finally find a parking spot, but someone cuts you off and grabs it. Or you find out you just won the lottery. These two different situations bring out two different emotions, and recognizing those emotions is the self-awareness part. The self-regulation part is how you react. Are you going to ram your car into the other one, or run down the driver when he gets out? Of course not. You may feel like it, but you will probably control yourself by counting to ten or doing some car yoga, and then just look for another spot.

Many children on the spectrum suffer from sensory overload. It is also difficult for them to understand what they are feeling and how to control their emotional response. This is something that needs to be taught to them.

Various methods could be used to help them become more self-aware over time, to recognize when they are approaching sensory or emotional overload, and to communicate the need for a break. As they get older, giving them more responsibility for scheduling their own breaks and choosing their own appropriate coping strategies can be very empowering.

Here are some tips on teaching self-regulation:

- Work on teaching self-awareness by teaching her to recognize emotion in others and herself. Pictures of different facial expressions that also show the feelings another person is exhibiting (i.e., a baby crying) are very useful for explaining emotion. Talking about your feelings and helping identify how she might be feeling also promotes self-awareness.
- If a person is prone to emotional or sensory overload, help her learn how to recognize what her "tipping" point is before she reaches it. At first, you will be the one to recognize it. When she is calm, use social stories to explain what you saw as the tipping point, and have her identify what she was feeling.
- Once she can recognize her tipping point, teach her to use a "break" card before she reaches the point of no return.
- Respect her need for a break.
- Teach her to use breathing or counting techniques.

- Teach her to have an item that helps her stay calm—a ball she can squeeze, a piece of ribbon in her pocket, or a book to look at.

Self-regulation can be taught using different techniques but starts with self-awareness.

Why don't they look me in the eye?

There is much discussion about eye contact and whether it is something we should insist that people with autism should learn as it does not come naturally to them. Eye contact is very important to neurotypicals because it indicates that the person you are speaking with is paying attention to what you have to say. When making eye contact, neurotypicals can pick up on nonverbal cues from the person they are making contact with.

Again, the answer as to whether we need to insist upon eye contact is not a simple one and should be treated on an individual basis. Many educators and parents of children and teens on the more able end of the spectrum may feel it is important to ensure that the person appears as neurotypical as possible.

What is it that makes it hard for those on the spectrum to look you in the eye? For one thing, they are not wired to pick up on the emotional or nonverbal cues the rest of us do when making eye contact. Also, many on the spectrum report that they are mono-channel, meaning that if they are visually processing information, they cannot process what is said. So a person may be staring at your eyes and focusing on how many millimeters your pupils changed, but won't have processed a thing you said.

Some on the spectrum report that they do not process a whole face when looking at someone, but instead see a Picasso-type painting with the eyes, nose, and mouth as jagged pieces of a puzzle, unrelated to one other and moving around. They become mesmerized by all the weird things moving, not realizing someone is talking to them.

The question is, what is the purpose or goal of teaching someone to make eye contact? If it is in hopes they will pick up the social cues, it is important to look at the individual to see if they have mastered learning all the body language cues we take for granted, because cues from eye contact are the most subtle, complex, and difficult to learn. If a person has been unable to learn the other kinds of nonverbal cues, there is a fair chance he will be unable to learn the subtleties of eye contact social cues.

If the goal is to make the person appear more neurotypical and make others more comfortable around him, then eye contact is important in situations—attending college, working, being out in the community—in which people expect eye contact to build and maintain relationships. One way of handling this is to teach the person with autism to stare at the top of the other person's ear. The person he is conversing with will think that he is looking him in the eye, and the person on the spectrum is still able to focus on the conversation.

If the reason is to ensure that the person is paying attention and hearing what is said, it is better to let them look where it is more comfortable for them so they can focus on listening. You can always check by asking a few questions to see whether they have been listening and processing what has been said.

Eye contact usually serves no purpose for a person on the spectrum, and to insist on eye contact can be detrimental to their focusing on the conversation.

Why are emotions hard for them to understand?

Just as many on the spectrum have a hard time identifying what their body is feeling in terms of physical needs (not knowing whether discomfort in the stomach area means they are hungry or their bladder is full), they also have a hard time understanding the emotions they are feeling.

Many neurotypicals assume that those on the spectrum do not feel emotions. This is far from the truth. Many with Asperger's have shared that they believe this assumption goes back to their communication difficulties and the major difference in the way they communicate emotions. It is not natural for people on the spectrum to communicate their emotions in a social context the way that it appears to be for neurotypicals. For those on the spectrum, it requires much effort and energy. Some with motor planning difficulties report not being able to move their facial muscles to show the emotions they are feeling.

As children, we learn to recognize emotional states because we observe the people around us. We learn that a smile means happy and crying means sad, and we then relate those emotions to how we are feeling. Eventually we become aware of what we are feeling and what those feelings mean; this is developing self-awareness. Usually children on the spectrum do not pick up this information about feelings by watching others because they are not good at deciphering body language and facial cues.

Adults with autism report that because of the difficulties of recognizing the emotions they are feeling, they cannot know what steps to take to get rid of the particular feeling, such as loneliness. Often, overwhelming emotions can lead to emotional overload, much like sensory overload.

Some tips on how to help someone on the spectrum identify and handle emotions:

- What emotions look like on someone's face can be taught through the use of modeling, photos, and videos. Identify for them what particular facial expressions indicate, like "That baby is crying because he is hungry," or "I am sad Grandma is sick, and that is why the corners of my mouth are turned down."
- Over time, helping them understand the emotions they are feeling ("You have tears running down your face, so you are probably feeling sad inside") will help them become self-aware.
- Teaching them to identify the emotional triggers, and what they can do to prevent or diffuse them so as not to have an emotional overload, is necessary to help them with self-regulation.

Helping them identify what emotions look like on others and on themselves can help them understand the feelings they have and prevent emotional overload.

How can we teach them self-esteem and self-advocacy?

Self-esteem, or confidence in one's own abilities, is a necessary precursor to a happy adult life. It is clear that those who appear self-confident and have good self-esteem tend to have had a few things in common while growing up. Adults I interviewed on this topic related that the most important factor was parents or caretakers who were accepting of their child, yet expected them to reach their potential and sought out ways to help them. Kamran Nazeer, author of *Send in the Idiots: Stories from the Other Side of Autism*, explained that having a relationship with an adult who was more neutral than parents and not as emotionally involved was important as well. Parents naturally display a sense of expectations, while a teacher, mentor, or therapist can be supportive of a child and accepting of the behavioral and social challenges. Relationships with non-autistic peers, as well as autistic peers who share the same challenges, were also important in developing confidence.

Tips to help a person develop good self-esteem:

- Always speak in front of the person as if they understand; nonverbal does not mean non-hearing and non-understanding.
- What they hear is what they believe. Speak positively about them because everything you say makes an impact on the person listening.
- Respect their wishes. Give them choices, ask their opinions, and then respect those choices by following through.

Having good self-esteem is necessary for learning how to advocate for oneself. To be able to self-advocate, a person has to have self-confidence. Self-advocacy is a necessary skill for all ability levels, and is important in the IEP process. Legally a student must give input about their IEP starting at age fourteen or sixteen, depending on the state. How he or she gives that input may look different for each person depending on their ability level.

The issue of disclosure concerning a diagnosis is a heated one with parents, teachers, and adults on the spectrum. "Should we or should we not disclose, to whom and how?" is one of the questions I get asked most at my presentations.

To be effective, self-advocacy entails a certain amount of disclosure. Some believe in full disclosure to all, while others choose to disclose only the area of difficulty. All the adults I spoke with believed all children should be told about their diagnosis, and in a positive manner. Adults with autism also appreciated learning of their diagnosis. Michael John Carley, who was diagnosed following the diagnosis of his son, says he always felt different than others. For him, his diagnosis was liberating because then he knew why he felt different.

Some tips for teaching self-advocacy:

- Giving choices within parameters to a young child on the spectrum, and respecting her choices, is a good way to start teaching self-advocacy. Children first rely on their parents, and little by little, they learn to order in a restaurant, then to tell a shopkeeper what they are looking for, ask a teacher for help, or stick up for themselves when they are being picked on by classmates. Even those severely impacted by autism need to be able to make their wants and needs known. Making even basic choices is a starting point for self-advocacy.

- Teaching assertiveness is important. Being able to protect oneself from an invasion of privacy is an essential safety skill that begins with assertiveness, and is, in effect, the first step towards being able to self-advocate. For example, teaching a child to independently order food in a restaurant and to clarify what he or she wants (with or without assistive technology for those who have limited verbal skills) is one way of teaching appropriate assertiveness. Kassiane Alexandra Sibley, who wrote a chapter in the book *Ask and Tell,* offers the example of a child who is light sensitive and thus unable to focus or learn in the classroom. By using a mentor or facilitator, a young student can learn to approach the teacher about possible solutions when she is experiencing a difficulty, such as a light sensitivity.

- Children who are fully included in general education have an even greater need early on to be aware of the sensory challenges they face so that they can learn to ask for accommodations instead of having meltdowns due to sensory issues in the classrooms when a teacher may have no clue what is going on. For this to happen, children have to have a sufficient amount of self-awareness and mentors they can model who will help them reach a point at which they can advocate for themselves. For more information on self-esteem and self-advocacy, read *Autism Life Skills.*

Learning to advocate for himself has been tremendous for my son's self-esteem, but has also put him in the position of taking more responsibility for his behavior and for communicating in an appropriate manner. And isn't that our hope for all teenagers—on or off the spectrum?

Self-esteem and self-advocacy both involve self-awareness. Good self-esteem can be instilled by the way people are treated by those they know, and self-advocacy can be taught through small steps and with the help of a mentor.

What are the thirteen things to know about raising and educating a teenager on the spectrum?

Often, I get e-mails from parents and educators about the children with autism they know who are just becoming teenagers. "Help," they write. "His autism is getting worse; what should I do?" I am lucky because I have raised two teenagers, one on the spectrum and another who is neurotypical, and this has given me a greater perspective on the matter. The reality is that their autism is not getting worse—they are simply becoming teenagers!

Besides becoming more noncompliant, major challenges with any teenager is that sometime during the teen years, most of them become uncommunicative, moody, unwilling to spend time with you, and never willing to do what you want to do.

When tweens with autism go through puberty and hit the teen years, they also have the same hormonal activity taking place as neurotypical teens, only they don't have the same outlets as neurotypicals to express their teenagehood.

When I give seminars on autism and adolescence, I like to remind people a few facts about teenage behavior—on or off the autism spectrum—to put things into perspective. Here is my Top Thirteen Things Every Person Needs to Know About Teenagers:

13. Teenage behavior cannot be blamed on mercury, vaccinations, or the parents' genetics.
12. Some teenagers care about smelling good. Or not.
11. Some like orderliness. Or not.
10. Teenagers do not learn self-esteem by themselves.
9. Teenagers like to make their own choices. They are not usually the same as yours.
8. Teenagers do not learn develop good organizational skills through osmosis.
7. Moodiness is a normal teenage state of mind.
6. Raging hormones are part of being a teenager.
5. Self-regulation is an important life skill not practiced by teenagers.
4. Teenagers are never hungry at the same time as the rest of the family.
3. Masturbation is normal teenage activity.
2. Discussing sex with your parents is not.
1. As a parent, you will survive the teen years. Barely.

Here are some tips to help you and your teen on the spectrum not only survive the adolescent years, but to grow in a positive way:

- Allow the teen to be noncompliant in appropriate ways. Noncompliance in a teen on the spectrum is harder to handle than with neurotypical teens (addressed in the following chapter).
- Teach your teen to perform chores. Teens need to learn that living with other people entails responsibilities as well as pleasures. Depending on the ability level of the teen, there are different ways in which he can contribute to the household.

- Explain to your child about his or her changing body. Imagine how scary it must be to realize your body is going through some strange metamorphosis and you don't know why, and yet there is nothing you can do about it. This is especially difficult for those who do not like change.
- Watch out for seizures. One out of every four teenagers with autism will develop seizures during puberty. Although the exact reason is unknown, this seizure activity may be due to hormonal changes in the body. For many, the seizures are small and subclinical, not typically detected by simple observation. Some signs that a teen may be experiencing subclinical seizures include making little or no academic gains after doing well during childhood and preteen years, losing some behavioral or cognitive gains, or exhibiting behavior problems such as self injury, aggression, and severe tantruming that do not appear to have an antecedent or pattern.
- Teach your child that masturbation is a private activity. It's going to take place no matter what you do, so the best approach is to teach your teen that this is an activity to be done in private. Designate a private place in the home (his bedroom) as the only place this activity may be allowed. If masturbation is occurring at school, it should not be allowed. The student should be redirected and told he can have private time at home. This necessitates good communication between home and school.
- Relationships and sexuality are topics that need discussing. It is necessary to talk to your teen on the spectrum about sex and the many types of relationships that exist between people. No matter the functioning level of your child, he or she needs to know about appropriate and inappropriate greetings, touch, and language.
- Teens out in the community on their own need to learn the rules that cannot be broken in terms of appropriate behavior in public. Otherwise, they risk getting into trouble and getting arrested.

- Parents, take time out. Whether you take a short break every day to take a walk, exercise, or engage in a favorite activity, or a weekly evening out at with your significant other, you need to recharge your batteries. This is also positive modeling for your teen or preteen, teaching them that although life can be stressful for all of us, we need to find ways to manage our stress and enjoy life.

For parents and educators who need more in-depth information, read *Adolescents on the Autism Spectrum* and visit Autism College at http://autismcollege.com.

Autism and adolescence together can form a volatile mix, but with some explaining and strategies in place, it becomes a time of positive growth.

Why do preteens and teens have a hard time with the body changes that puberty brings?

Many children on the autism spectrum have a terrible time with change. They like things to stay the same, as they are used to the familiarity of routine. If there are no new things, they don't have to anticipate any "attacks" to their senses; they can anticipate what is coming next. Many like things to be the same and will spend time lining up their toys or objects. Some parents have reported that when they have moved the furniture around, the child would move it back to where it used to be.

Now, imagine that you are the type of person who cannot stand change, that you are afraid of it. And then you notice something really freaky—your body is changing, and you have no control over it. It is even worse if no one has told you what was going to happen. Boys start noticing the hair on their legs growing in tougher and longer, and hair sprouting in places there wasn't any before. Then, they notice their Adam's apple has grown and become more prominent, and their voice is starting to change and is cracking at times. Not only that, but something weird is happening "down there."

For girls, it is much the same; think of all the ways a girl's body changes, and imagine how frightful that could be if you don't like change. Especially when the girl begins to menstruate, if no one has explained to her in a way she can understand what that is all about, then she will have a difficult time going through this change towards womanhood.

Some tips:

- It is best to start explaining to the preteen what bodily changes to expect before puberty hits. However, better late than never. For girls, puberty usually starts at age nine or ten, for boys at ten or eleven.
- Explain what will happen to both the male and female bodies during puberty, so that the child is not surprised when they see their peers changing as well.
- Show pictures of trusted, loved adults of both sexes—mom, dad, aunt, uncle—as babies, then children, then teens, then as adults, so that they see how the transformation has happened to everyone, and that it is a positive thing to go through.
- Explain the bodily functions inherent to being a boy and being a girl. If you have a girl on the spectrum, it might be a wise idea to have her wear a pad for a while before she begins her menstrual cycles, so that she gets used to the sensory aspect of wearing the sanitary pad.
- The use of social stories and a picture book you can create with the above information is helpful. You can then go over the picture book and social stories as often as needed.

For more information on puberty and hygiene, read *Adolescents on the Autism Spectrum*.

Body changes are scary for those who do not like change,
but telling and showing them the changes that will happen can
make it much easier.

Why does it seem like their autism is getting worse at puberty?

Something happens when children turn into teenagers. They go from demanding your attention to wanting their independence. For those on the spectrum, it may look like noncompliance; they don't seem to want to follow through on your requests anymore. As a parent it may be hard to appreciate, but this is a necessary development. Being appropriately noncompliant is a positive step towards self-advocacy. However, it is important to differentiate between appropriate teenage noncompliance and problem behaviors that must be stopped. It's also important to support your teen as he struggles to become his own person.

When tweens on the spectrum go through puberty and hit the teen years, they also have the same hormones acting up as the neurotypical teens, and they feel the need to be more independent, only they don't have the same outlets as neurotypicals to show their independence. Thus we see more defiant and noncompliant behavior.

Neurotypical teens are able to communicate to us that they need independence, more time away from their parents, and more choice over how they will spend their time. Sometimes they start acting up by staying out later than a pre-established curfew, going to parties, and getting into environments where they have to make choices about their behavior. They start negotiating with us to change house rules in regards to their social outings. At school, they are involved in small group projects or on sports teams and get to make choices that affect the team.

For example, my daughter, Rebecca, loves alternative rock concerts, and had been asking to attend them since she was 11 years old. When she was in high school, the rules changed in regards to attending concerts. When she was 11, she could go on a weekend night with a few friends if there was a trusted parent who stayed with them the whole time, and if she was home at a certain time. At 17, she was allowed to stay out later, did not have to have an adult accompany her, and at times could go during the week, depending on school and her sport schedule. The rules changed because as she got older, Rebecca argued her case to us about why she should be allowed to stay out later, and she had demonstrated responsibility.

Preteens and teens with autism, however, usually don't negotiate or tell their parents they need more space, even if they are verbal. They rarely have opportunities outside the home with other teens that are testing their parents' authority. Yet they have the same hormones and the same urge to have more freedom. This leads to noncompliance, which is never any fun for those involved.

So, how can we as parents and educators provide them more freedom and space? Here are some tips:

- Give him more opportunities to make choices, within parameters. For example, if a teenager has had a schedule to stick to after school, why not give him the choice of what order to do it in?
- At school, provide more opportunities for making choices, perhaps in choosing the group activity, or more control over planning his schedule, and in how he spends his day.

- Give him the choice of what the family will eat for dinner (within limits) once or twice a week. Maybe he can even do the shopping and help prepare the meal. This can help him learn responsibility as well.
- Instead of always planning activities or outings for your teen on the weekends, pick one day where your teen can choose on a regular basis what his afternoon will look like.

Noncompliance is normal teenage activity, not exclusive to teens on the spectrum.

Are adults on the spectrum interested in long-term relationships, marriage, and sex?

Many on the spectrum are interested in dating and marriage, yet these types of personal relationships are challenging for them. The difficulty they have in recognizing emotions in themselves and others, as well as the communication difficulties they have, can lead to ongoing challenges in those relationships, both big and small. The inability to communicate about what they are feeling can cause people with Asperger's to be perceived as uncaring or as lacking accountability, although the reality may be the opposite. In situations in which they know they have acted in a way they let their partner down, they may be internally beating themselves up, but just don't know how to communicate it, make it right, or how to comfort the other person. Put simply, they are at a loss as to how to act.

The emotional processing and communications issues can wreak havoc on a person's ability to build and sustain adult relationships. However, awareness of why these issues happen can make a big difference in relationships.

Even for those on the autism spectrum, dating can be awkward and mystifying. The challenges of beginning as acquaintances and then becoming friends and then perhaps a significant other requires good communication skills—verbal, nonverbal, and pragmatic—which are not easy for someone on the spectrum.

Some of those on the more impacted end of the spectrum have also communicated their wish for more involvement with others, yet have even more difficulties than those with Asperger's. For those with motor planning difficulties, the sexual aspect of personal relationships may seem nearly impossible. There are many who crave the closeness of sexual intimacy, but because of sensory sensitivities may have difficulties in this area.

So by looking at what could make socialization and dating easier for non-spectrum people and by boosting the amplitude some, perhaps it is possible to arrive at accommodations that will not only be useful to those on the spectrum, but perhaps assist a larger population of people too.

Stephen Shore, a well-known author on the spectrum who is married, has these observations on developing personal relationships:

- People on the spectrum are not good at chitchat, so the communication needs to be more direction-oriented. Activity-based gatherings, such as school clubs based on a common interest (music, chess, computers), are much easier for those on the spectrum than socially intensive activities like going to a bar.
- There are three types of dates that each serve a purpose: play dates (based on shared interest), homework dates (working on an activity together), and serious dates (establishing a more personal connection).
- It is important to help teens or young adults identify the social cues and body language in neurotypicals that signals an interest in dating.
- Ensuring that young people are not getting bullied at school and helping the person to learn to advocate for himself is helpful for relationship building.

- Marriage requires good and direct communication in order to understand why a partner may do something (for example, Stephen hid a clock that his wife needed for practicing her harp because the ticking was too painful and annoying to him).

Stephen also shares these tips on how parents can help their child with autism develop the skills he or she needs to build any relationship, from friendship to romance:

- Learn more about the subtleties of adolescence and relationships. Find resources that you find most comfortable: on the Internet, books, from other parents, educators, counselors, and so on.
- Encourage your child to get involved with activities of interest that involve interacting with others in group or clublike settings. The interaction with others will then be based on the activity or interest at hand, without the pressure of social interaction being the main reason for getting together.
- Teach your teens and young adults how to interact with others when a romantic interest is present. It is important that they learn the importance of not forcing oneself on another and are able to recognize a lack of interest on the part of the other. There are many more issues related to dating, and finding appropriate resources is helpful. Reading the experiences of adults on the spectrum can provide insight on how to help your child.

For more information, read *A Full Life with Autism* and visit Autism College at http://autismcollege.com.

Many on the spectrum do want personal long-term relationships, but because of difficulties in communication and with emotions, becoming involved with another person can be problematic. However, parents can help prepare their teens and young adults.

What is college like for young adults on the spectrum?

College can be a great experience for someone on the spectrum. A college is a mini society that some like so much they stay on as professors. For others, it can be overwhelming. Some may be adjusting to a new living situation as well as a new school and new schedule. While in high school, he may have had a full day's school schedule already worked out and only had to concern himself with organizing his afterschool and weekend schedule. Now at college, he may have classes a few times a week and a lot more independent work to complete. Planning over time is not a skill that comes naturally to people on the spectrum, so sometimes this can cause the student to fall way behind in coursework. Also, work cannot be modified at the college level, and the student, not the parent, must request any accommodations. Social connections in a new environment may not be obvious.

However, there are many ways we can prepare high school students headed for college. Here are some tips:

- Make sure that while your child is still in high school, he learns the executive functions he will need to survive as a more independent adult. The executive functions have to do with managing time, planning, and getting and staying organized.

- Help him figure out a system that works for him to keep and stay organized. This could mean color coding subject books and notebooks, filing systems, and so on.
- If he likes technology, he can use computers and handheld calendars and similar tools to keep track of projects and plan out when he needs to do certain steps for each school project.
- Ensure he learns to schedule his free time so that when he has gaps of unscheduled times, the time is not wasted, that he knows what to do and what to work on.
- As a student he will need to learn how to ask for his own accommodations. This means he needs to learn how to identify the accommodation he needs and how to self-advocate for it. The IEP process is a good way for him to learn how to do this.
- If your child will be away at college, make sure you have a mutually agreed-upon communication schedule with him. Many parents report being concerned about not having heard from their child and assume the worst. Often, those with Asperger's do not like communicating on the phone and do not understand the need to keep in touch. Explain the rationale behind a twice-a-week phone call—it lets the parents know their child is okay and that the child will know everything is okay at home.
- If your child will be going away to college, make sure he has a schedule of when to do his laundry and keep his room in order, and what having a roommate entails in terms of responsibility and communication.
- Ensure that he has hooked into the clubs or groups that relate to his areas of interest. He can create a social network based on mutual passions.

For more information, read *A Full Life with Autism* and visit Autism College at http://autismcollege.com.

College can be an exciting but scary time for someone on the spectrum. Learning executive function skills can help that person adjust.

Why is it so hard for adults with autism to find and keep a job?

It is hard for adults on the spectrum to find and keep a job for a variety of reasons, starting with the challenges they face in the areas of communication, social relationships, and their passionate interest in usually one area of focus. Add in the lack of employer awareness about autism, and lack of knowledge of many job coaches on specific strategies to help support a person on the job, and all this makes for a high unemployment rate for those on the spectrum, including those with Asperger's.

Unemployment rates for working-age adults with disabilities in 2002 hovered around the seventy percent rate for the twelfth year in a row, according to the 2002 Report from the President's Commission on Excellence in Special Education. This report suggests we were not doing a good enough job of preparing our teenagers and young adults in transition programs for life as working adults. Since then, mandates in regards to transition services under IDEA have been strengthened, and hopefully we are now doing a better job of preparing our youth.

In my interviews of adults on the spectrum, some adults I

spoke with struggled for years before finding an area they could work in. The life skills discussed previously tremendously impact a person's ability to find, get, and keep a job.

Temple Grandin, who co-authored the book *Developing Talents*, says that parents should help their children develop their natural talents, and that young people need mentors to give them guidance and valuable experience. Authors John Elder Robison (*Look Me in the Eye*) and Daniel Tammet (*Born on a Blue Day*) both credit their Asperger's for giving them the talents on which they have based their successful businesses. What parents and teachers see as "obsessive interests" when a child on the spectrum is passionate about a topic can actually become something they can base a career on or earn money doing. For example, when younger, author and advocate Stephen Shore used to take apart timepieces and put them back together again. Years later, this interest was translated into paid work repairing bicycles at a bike store.

For those whose talents are less obvious, a look at the community they live in and the service needs that exist there could create an opportunity to earn money. My son, Jeremy, and his teacher created a sandwich-delivering business and then a flower-selling business on his high school campus as part of his work experience. Customized employment, including self-employment, with careful planning and implementation could be a solution for some.

Some of the skills discussed in this book, such as self-regulation, independence, social relationships, and self-advocacy, are important for getting and keeping a job. Being able to get and hold a job is really a culmination of all the life skills learned during the school-age years, whether a person is on or off the spectrum. For example, for someone to be accepted in a workplace, they must be able to control their emotional and sensory meltdowns. And a certain amount of independence is needed at most jobs. Understanding that you should speak to your boss differently than you would to a colleague is important to know in most work situations. Self-advocacy skills are necessary in order to request what you need to get the job done.

Here are some tips for helping a person find and keep a job:

- Life skills in general should be broken down and translated into IEP goals and objectives, especially during middle school, high school, and transitional years. Obviously, everyone is different, and the skill level reached will be different depending on the person; but every student needs to learn a minimum of these skills in order to live and work in the community.

- Look at the top skills employers look for in an employee, and focus on "selling" the prospective employer on the points the prospective employee has. The point is, when people are selling a product or service, they market the positive attributes, not the negatives. And that's precisely what we need to be doing with any prospective employees on the spectrum. For example, honesty and a strong work ethic are two positive attributes most on the spectrum have, and they are the two highest attributes wanted by employers.

  Those on the spectrum may find helpful the list of the top ten skills and attributes most employers look for as identified by the Bureau of Labor Statistics (*Job Outlook*, 2003): honesty and integrity; a strong work ethic; analytical skills; computer skills; teamwork; time management and organizational skills; communication skills (oral and written); flexibility; interpersonal skills; and motivation/initiative. An individual will increase his likelihood of obtaining a job if he can promote a skill or attribute he has from this list.

- Consider what your child or student likes or is passionate (obsessed) about, and figure out how that can help him earn money. In most cases, people on the spectrum can be difficult to motivate—unless it involves something they are really into. The trick is to figure out how to use that interest and turn it into a moneymaker, or to find a career field that can use that particular interest or talent.

- Make a list of the strengths and weaknesses that the prospective employee has. This will be useful for narrowing down potential employment to some particular job areas. Looking at organization skills, whether the person likes to work indoors or outdoors, likes to move around or stay in one place, and likes routine or change are all important things to consider when trying to make a match.

- There are different employment structures currently available. By analyzing a person's strengths and weaknesses and likes and dislikes, and by asking some of the questions above, a clearer idea of what could be a good match with the person on the spectrum is possible. There is full-time work, part-time employment, seasonal work, year-round employment, and more.

- Mentors can help figure out how to turn an interest into a job, or into a means to earn money. Temple Grandin (*Thinking in Pictures, Developing Talents*) speaks often about the importance of mentors in helping to turn interests into marketable skills. She had mentors from her science teacher at school to her aunt, family friends, and colleagues. Guidance from these people is what helped her become the success she is today. If your child appears to have skills or a real interest in a specific area, someone who works in that field can help the child realize the application of his interests. Parents may realize their child's talent but not know about a certain area of employment related to that talent.

- Other less traditional structures are becoming more popular, including customized employment, which means the work is tailored to the individual, not the other way around. It can entail job carving, in which one job is carved up into different tasks shared by several people, giving each employee the part of the job they enjoy or excel at the most. Another type of customized employment is self-employment, sometimes referred to as micro-enterprise.

- Those with specific skills need to have an effective visual portfolio (drawings, cover letter, articles) to "wow" the interviewer, as people on the spectrum tend to do poorly in interviews.

The future is more hopeful as people are coming up with more creative solutions to the unemployment situation. For example, Thorkil Sonne, a pioneering dad in Denmark, has created a company called Specialisterne that helps people with autism and Asperger's syndrome find employment in the computer tech industry. This is a great model of how to integrate highly talented yet misunderstood people into the workforce.

For more information on jobs and autism, read *A Full Life with Autism* and visit Autism College at http://autismcollege.com.

Teaching life skills, analyzing the needs of the potential employee and employer, looking at different employment structures, and finding mentors can help with a successful transition to employment.

What hope is there for the future for people on the autism spectrum?

Thirty years ago, I worked with young adults who were preparing to leave the state hospital they knew as home, for a more inclusive life in group homes in the community. The future for people on the spectrum looks brighter in many ways than it did then.

The specialist who diagnosed Jeremy when he was three years old gave me a box of pencils and said, "If you are lucky, you will find a good institution for your son. He will eventually learn to package pencils into a box. That's where these came from." teen years later, I found an institution: it's called College. That is where my son headed after he graduated from high school. This would never have been possible thirty years ago. My son's success is not a result of any miracle. It is the result of much blood, sweat, and tears (on his part and mine) and the hard work of many educators, home tutors, and myself.

A few years ago, Jeremy was highlighted on the MTV documentary series *True Life* in the award-winning episode "I Have Autism." The documentary followed Jeremy around his high

school and community and showed him learning to use an assistive technology device to have a voice, and making friends and
connecting with his peers. This, too, would never have been possible a couple of decades ago.

Why am I more hopeful that my son's future as an adult will
be different than those young adults I worked with thirty years
ago? Here are some reasons:

- Children are being diagnosed at a much earlier age, so intervention can start earlier to help them.
- Biomedical interventions are available to help those with
medical issues.
- There are more support groups in place to help families trying to figure out what is best to do for their child.
- There is more community acceptance and changed attitudes toward differently-abled people.
- More laws are in place to guarantee and protect the rights
of people like my son.
- There are more treatments, therapies, and strategies we can
use to help people on the spectrum.
- Autism advocates are pushing for and getting health-cov-
erage laws passed in many states to ensure that insurance
companies will provide for treatment of children with autism.
- More money than ever before is being spent on research
into different causes, effective treatments, best practices in
education, and the best practices in programs and supports
for adults.
- Nonprofit organizations and state and federal agencies are
working together to create and assist with housing and employment for adults.

But perhaps the biggest change is the growing field of neuroplasticity. Not too long ago, the brain was believed to be hardwired
and incapable of fundamental change. Not anymore. Science has

now come to appreciate the brain's plasticity, and they believe that if one pathway gets blocked, the brain can find alternative pathways. We know that the brain is capable of developing new and more appropriate circuitry in a process called neuroplasticity. This means that the window of opportunity for learning never closes, and there is always hope that, even as adults, people on the spectrum can continue to learn what they need to live content lives. It also means that neurotypical people can learn to be more supportive and accepting of others who are not so unlike us after all.

Although there are many challenges in meeting everyone's needs, there is much hope for the future as parents, nonprofit organizations, and the government work hard to solve the mysteries of autism, and create a brighter future.

CPSIA information can be obtained at www.ICGtesting.com
Printed in the USA
BVOW070847150312

285269BV00001B/2/P